AN APPLE A DAY:

Collective Wisdom for Your Body and Soul

An Anthology Brought to You by
Gift an Author Publishing

GIFT AN AUTHOR PUBLISHING, LLC

DENTON, TEXAS

An Apple a Day: Collective Wisdom for Your Body and Soul

Compiled and Published by Gift An Author Publishing, LLC

Copyright © 2025 by Gift An Author Publishing, LLC. All rights reserved.

ISBN-13:

- Paperback: 978-1-968445-06-5

- Hardback: 978-1-968445-05-8

- eBook978-1-968445-07-2

Published by: Gift An Author Publishing, LLC 5405 Zara Drive Denton, Texas 72607

Library of Congress Cataloging-in-Publication Data

Printed in the United States of America and China

First Edition

TABLE OF CONTENTS

WHY THIS BOOK WAS BORN

Kristine Skiff, CEO Gift an Author Publishing

There was a time when I could no longer feel my own tears.

I sat in a doctor's office with my twelve-year-old, hearing yet another life-altering diagnosis—this time, schizoaffective disorder—and as the words landed in the air, something wet dropped onto my hand. I looked up, confused, checking the ceiling for a leak. But there was no leak.

I was crying.

After years of managing specialists, therapies, medications, and mountains of paperwork for all five of my children—each of whom had been diagnosed in early childhood with autism and later with mental health conditions like bipolar disorder, severe anxiety, and more—I had become so efficient, so pragmatic, so relentlessly "on," that I didn't recognize the tears on my own skin.

My husband had been diagnosed as autistic during our children's diagnostic process, then later with MS and bipolar disorder. My life was consumed by caregiving, navigating the complex systems of health and mental wellness for everyone in my family. I had learned to take the blows with grace. I became skilled at carrying the weight of it all. I wore resilience like armor.

Until that day in the doctor's office, when the armor cracked.

It was my friends who insisted I go to therapy. It was my therapist who helped me reconnect to my own body, who taught me to pause every twenty minutes and ask:

Am I clenching my jaw?

Is my stomach in knots?

Have I been sighing without noticing?

And slowly, breath by breath, I began to find myself again—not in grand epiphanies, but in the smallest of awarenesses. I learned to breathe again. I learned to listen to my body. I learned to feel what I had numbed out in service to others. That was the beginning of my journey toward natural healing and holistic wellness—a journey that would take me through Buddhist and Hindu traditions, through writing, through breathwork, and eventually to starting a publishing company where I could amplify the voices of others doing deep healing work.

One of the most honest things I've ever written came from that era, when my youngest child's diagnosis cracked my soul open. I wrote:

Words, I have a deep and abiding love for words... all words.

Words and I have been best friends for as long as I can remember. My mother often talks about just how early words found me.

Indeed, I love everything about words; the musical lilt of the vowels and consonance as they trip off the tongue, the little shiver that runs down my spine when the words meet to form a perfect, balanced and beautiful sentence.

But what happens when the words stop? When no matter how hard you try there are no words to cry, to scream, to whisper… there are just no words?

This is the deepest grief for me. Grief that has clawed my soul so deeply that it has stolen not only my voice but also my vocabulary.

To be fair, this grief is not a new grief; it has lived with me for a long time.

I didn't know that if you grieve long enough, you can burn out your soul.

I didn't know that you become so numb that you cease to feel grief at all.

But every camel has one last straw that will break its back, every bowl has a point at which it will overflow, and every heart has a point at which it cannot handle one more loss.

Then the day came, the doctor spoke the words, and then I broke; my breath caught and suddenly my words were gone.

This is what it is to burn out on grief.

This is what it is to lose your words.

This is what brokenness truly feels like.

© Kristine Skiff

That moment of voicelessness was the catalyst for everything that followed—for the healing, the curiosity, the breathwork, the blending of medicine and mindset, and ultimately for this book.

An Apple a Day is a love letter to every person who has ever put their own healing last.

It's a reminder that **you matter too**.

That **your voice deserves to be heard**.

And that sometimes, it just takes **one word** to begin again.

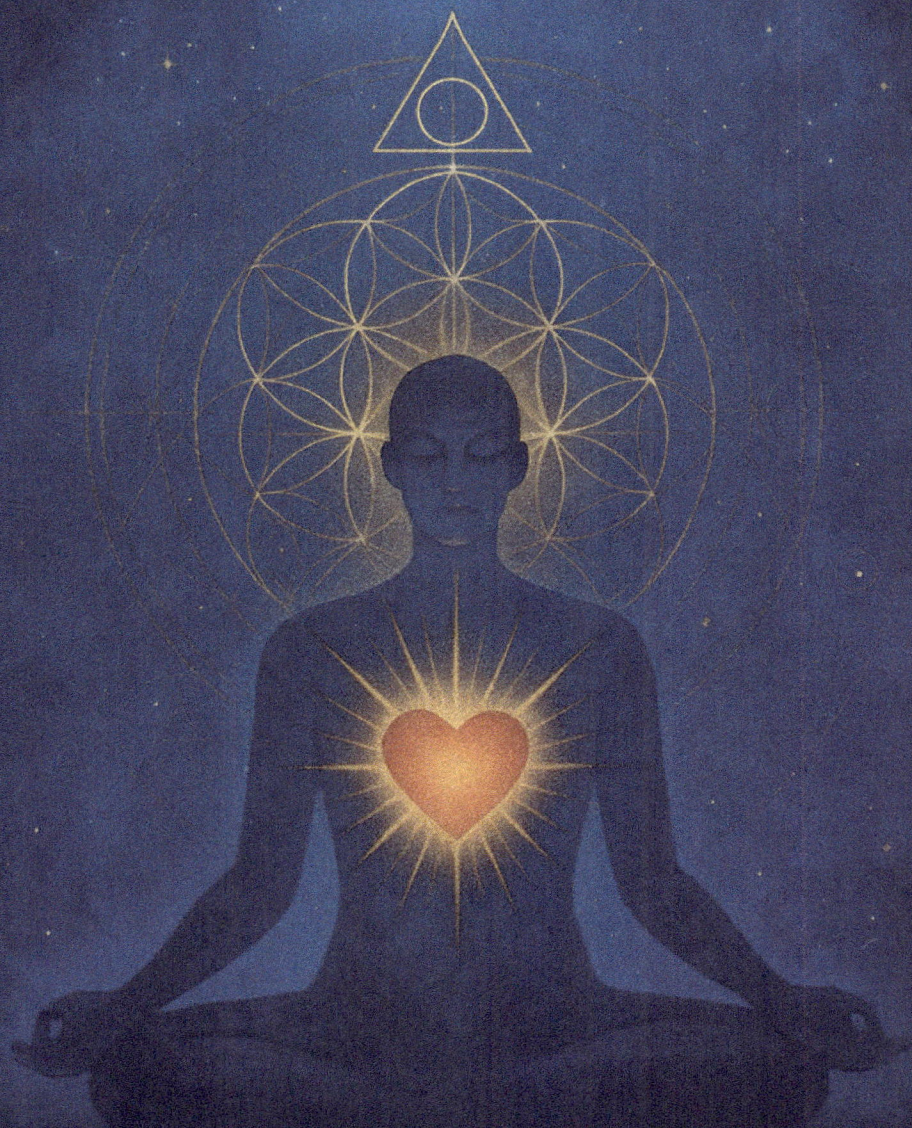

AWAKENING THE HEART

A JOURNEY OF DIVINE HEALING

CHAPTER ONE

AWAKENING THE HEART:

A JOURNEY OF DIVINE HEALING

Claudia Rocafort

In Loving Memory of Chantica Camejo,
dear friend and catalyst for my awakening,
and Railey Macey, thank you for Being
The Love, for awaking my heart, and for
showing me The Path to Oneness.

The moment I stepped into the Temple of Abydos in Egypt, it was as if the air itself recognized my soul. I had waited my whole life for this journey—drawn since childhood to the Egyptian temples, ancient gods, hieroglyphs, and myths with a pull I could never quite explain. But nothing could have prepared me for what happened that day.

As I crossed the threshold, I was engulfed in a sense of deep familiarity. The towering walls and majestic pillars seemed to embrace me, calling me inward. Deep inside the Inner Hall of Osiris, I had an unexpectedly vivid vision: I was standing there in another time, a pail of oil and flame in my hands, moving through the temple with purpose lighting sacred spaces in reverence to the divine. A priest dressed in leopard skin walked beside me anointing the statues of Isis and Osiris with precious scented oils. The scene unfolded like a vivid memory.

My heart pounded, my skin covered in goosebumps, my eyes filled with tears. It was a remembering--and with that remembering came a deep emotional recognition of why Egypt had always felt so close to my heart. I cried. I surrendered. I allowed myself to feel the sacredness and magnitude of the moment. And I realized that something profound connected me to this land—not just its history, but its mysticism.

That afternoon in the Temple of Dendera I saw myself again—as a young woman, around sixteen—traveling by boat to the Temple back when the Nile flowed directly to its grand entrance. There I saw myself as an apprentice, arriving to begin the sacred path of initiation to one day become a healer or a priestess, and life changed irrevocably in that instant as I *knew* that I had come home.

I finally understood why Egypt had been beckoning and whispering to my soul my whole life. It was no coincidence that this place had always called to me. There was something sacred here about rituals, healing, and spiritual truth that lived within me, too.

I had come full circle to my childhood fascination with Egypt—not just to experience in person the places I had studied for my Art History BA—but to awaken a part of myself I had forgotten.

This moment became the realization that a Divine Intelligence was guiding my path, opening a portal to a deeper truth about awakening the heart, healing, and the ancient wisdom that still beckons us today. That healing and remembering is what I will share with you in this chapter.

Heart Centered Healing

Heart Centered Healing is rooted in the belief that everything begins and ends in the heart. This concept is as old as the Ancient Egyptians, who believed the heart was the center of life. In modern times, growing interest in alternative and ancient medicines have become more prevalent, particularly since the 1980's, leading to the resurgence of Heart-Centered practices. Today, the term is widely used among Holistic practitioners to mean anything from Healing Touch Therapy and Reiki to a variety of energy healing modalities.

In modern culture, the heart has long been associated with our emotions. We believe it is where our deepest wounds reside and where our greatest healing takes place. One of the most transformative forms of healing I have ever experienced in my 38-year search was through a profound Heart Centered Healing Meditation taught by a master teacher who changed my life.

While the term 'Heart Centered Healing' is now often used to describe any practice that emphasizes compassion, love, or emotional presence, what I share in this chapter is a deeply guided process rooted in ancient universal principles, energetic alignment, and willing integration through meditation. Through this practice, I learned how to access, recognize, and clear, the limiting beliefs, energetic imprints, and unconscious patterns that keep us stuck—whether in our relationships, level of success, health, or sense of purpose. This work wasn't just about mindfulness or relaxation; it was about releasing, reprogramming, and realigning with the truth of who we are.

In this chapter, we will explore the principles behind this powerful healing modality, the habits that can magnify our wellbeing, and how our thoughts, emotions, and energetic frequencies shape not only our personal lives, but also the collective consciousness. By understanding these principles, we gain access to one of the most profound tools for healing and conscious creation: the awareness that when we heal ourselves, we also heal the world.

But before we dive into the principles behind this Heart Centered Healing Meditation, let me share a little of my journey with you—to illustrate why this work is so powerful and how it transformed my life from the inside out.

My journey into healing and personal development began after a life-changing car accident in my freshman year of pre-med studies. In an instant, my world was turned upside down, forcing me to confront not only the fragility of life but also the deeper questions of existence, purpose, and meaning. My physical recovery was only the beginning. The real work lay in understanding the layers of emotional, mental, and spiritual wounds that surfaced in the wake of that moment, and for years to come. It was a profound initiation into the power of the mind-body-spirit connection that altered my life path and led me deep into the world of healing, self-discovery, spirituality, and transformation.

Being confronted with mortality made me question everything, starting with WHY did I survive when my dearest childhood friend did not? The pursuit of a medical healing career shifted into looking for ways to feel alive in the present moment so that I could get through each day and understand the sadness and anger I was carrying. I transitioned into a theater major, began taking acting classes, performing with the college dance troupe, and studying psychology.

Acting and dance became both a lifeline and an avenue for healing. When I stepped onto a stage, I wasn't just playing a role—I was embodying the power of presence, the rawness of emotion, and the art of conscious expression. The craft demanded an intimate relationship with breath, a deep connection with my body, my feelings, awareness, and energy. I began to experience a symbiosis between these experiences as an outlet for personal healing. Every part of me was trying to process, release emotions, and heal through dance or by becoming a character that would allow me to express what I so desperately needed to, at a time when I didn't have the conscious awareness of what I was doing.

My passion for acting seamlessly wove itself into my spiritual journey, reinforcing the power of self-awareness, presence, the study of human behavior, expression, and the spoken word as tools for healing and transformation. I began to understand that HOW we communicate, both verbally and non-verbally, shapes our reality; it holds the power to create, to heal or harm—not just ourselves, but those around us.

Through the years, I also immersed myself in researching alternative healing, self-help, philosophy, metaphysics, religion, and ancient wisdom—not just to heal, but seeking to find answers, meaning, or purpose in life. I attended lectures and workshops with incredible teachers, including Deepak Chopra, Derek O'Neil, and a Course in Miracles with Marianne Williamson. I read all the new age books I could get my hands on in the 90s, hung out in the esoteric bookstores in NYC between auditions, and was introduced to the principles that govern our universe according to Hermetic philosophy through a profound book called The Kybalion.

In 2000, my path took a pivotal turn when I was introduced to an incredible master teacher, Railey Macey, whose Heart Centered Healing and meditation practices profoundly shaped my approach. What started as a personal session became a nine-year journey of studying, practicing, and ultimately integrating this powerful modality into every aspect of my life and work.

Those years of practice reshaped my understanding of healing, showing me that transformation is not just about fixing what is broken, but about remembering our truth and integrating our wholeness. The heart is not only the motor that keeps us alive but also our greatest teacher, our most powerful compass, and the center of creation. When we learn to operate from this space, everything shifts—our mindset, our relationships, our leadership, and ultimately our reality.

In 2006, I combined my experience on-camera and on-stage with what I had learned about the power of words into the corporate world by becoming a Communication

Consultant and Executive Coach, teaching Conscious Communication under the mentorship of Edmund Bingham. In 2016, I received my Certified Professional Coach credentials from the International Coaching Federation, became a Team Leader Coach during Covid training other coaches to achieve their certifications, added Career and Business Coaching to my repertory, and most recently got certified to facilitate the Rewired for Peace Trainings.

Through my personal journey, I discovered that the state of our physical and mental health is directly correlated with our mindset, and that true healing is not just physical but deeply connected to our emotional and spiritual well-being. This required mindfulness, self-reflection, and conscious decision-making—implementing daily rituals to address the needs of my mind, body, and spirit. The habits that contributed to my emotional recovery were: daily perspective shifts, journaling my feelings without judgement, time for meditation and reflection, weekly therapy or coaching, daily exercise (dance, walking or yoga), and shifting my mindset by choosing to look at the glass half full (vs half empty) and taking a stand for gratitude by focusing on three things I could be grateful for each day.

As I write this chapter and reflect on my journey, I realize that the times I have maintained these habits have become the most peaceful, joyful, and successful periods of my life. When

I forget these principles or stop implementing them because I let 'life take over', stress, anxiety, even depression can creep back in.

True well-being is not just about healing the past or working through the current challenges; it's about creating daily habits that support your vitality, balance, and fulfillment every day. Wellness is a journey—one mindful step, one nourishing practice, one empowered choice at a time.

Today, my work is a fusion of these influences—acting, communication, coaching, healing, and spiritual wisdom—finally blending my experience in personal development, leadership, and holistic wellness into my coaching practice. I am passionate about guiding others to align their mission-vision-&-purpose, giving clients the tools to uncover their Zone of Genius and align it with their career path, clearing the limiting beliefs that stop them from achieving their ultimate goals or fulfilling relationships, and providing the tools for them to heal for deep, lasting transformation, and self-realization.

So, let's dive right in to how this Heart Centered Healing Meditation can support YOU…

You may recall I mentioned that this work isn't just about mindfulness, love, or relaxation; it's about releasing, reprogramming, and realigning with the truth of who we are.

This brings us to the Law of Oneness—the foundation of this practice and the principle that everything in existence is interconnected.

The Law of Divine Oneness: A Universal Truth

The Law of Divine Oneness is a spiritual principle that underscores the interconnected nature of all things in the universe. It reveals that everything that exists, or will ever exist, is part of ONE WHOLE. This principle has been passed down through various cultures and spiritual traditions, with some of the earliest written examples found in Hermetic philosophy manuscripts from ancient Egypt and Greece over 2,000 years ago. The Law of Oneness is considered the first of the 7 Hermetic Principles and the foundation of the 12 Universal Laws, a set of intrinsic laws and unseen forces that govern the universe.

At its core, the Law of Oneness states that all things ever created originate from a singular Divine Source. If you were to imagine yourself as this Oneness, this Whole, the ALL— what many call God or Source or how I like to call it: GOD (the Grand Operating Design as Dr. John Dimartini calls it to remove religious connotations)—you would recognize that in such a state, there is no contrast, no duality. Without contrast, there is no light or dark, love or hate, beauty or ugliness, and there is no reference point from which GOD or The ALL can experience itself.

For the Oneness to experience itself, it had to fragment into creation: to separate itself into manifestation, polarity, duality, and gender. In doing so, each manifestation of the Oneness was given the opportunity to explore different facets of existence. Imagine this as a coin that can only know itself as a complete coin, and which can never experience heads or tails unless it separates from itself to observe the coin toss.

However, for the ALL to fully experience any aspect of itself objectively in creation or manifestation, ALL its creations must temporarily forget the truth of their Divine Origin and Divine Nature.

The Illusion of Separation and the Path to Reconnection

The Law of Oneness teaches that we are all connected to a Universal Consciousness. Through our inherent creative power and divine energy, our thoughts, actions, and emotions ripple out, influencing the world around us. This principle describes the interconnectedness of all things in the universe and emphasizes how everything—from the smallest atom to the vastest galaxies—is a manifestation and expression of the ALL.

The Law of Oneness explains how every individual, every situation, and every creation is connected to each other. What someone else thinks or does may affect your life in some unforeseen way—and vice versa—even if you are not aware of it, even when you don't know that it is happening at all. The Law of Oneness explains Quantum Physics, placebo effects, Déjà vu, intuition, and the myriads of unexplained phenomena in our universe.

Every person, being, animal, or energy in creation is an expression of the ALL. There is nothing that is not part of the Oneness, and no matter what it looks like, its source is the ALL—Divine Love and Divine Energy seeking to express itself.

Yet, as human beings, we often operate under the illusion of separation. We perceive ourselves as distinct from others, from nature, and from Source itself. This illusion is the root of misunderstanding, pain, suffering and war. In this illusion of separation, we forget that there is nothing outside of GOD or of the Oneness. That ALL of it is a part of us—of our Source of Being. In this illusion of separation, everything we experience as a dislike in another, is a part of ourselves that we are resisting or denying as part of the Oneness. When we reject any aspect of ourselves or another, we hold it as separate from Source. But in truth, all that we admire and all that we reject are simply reflections of different aspects of the Divine Oneness. The gift lies in recognizing the beliefs we are holding that are keeping us separate from the Divine creative nature and Divine Source that we are. We are all constant mirrors and regular beacons for each other to help us wake up from the illusion.

The greatest gift of the human experience is the realization that we are never truly separate. Each of us is an emanation of the Oneness, imbued with divine intelligence and with the power to create and manifest. We have chosen to "separate" from the Oneness into human form to experience more of the ALL that we are, to express and bear witness to the Infinite Facets of GOD. Our journey in this life is one of remembering, of embracing all aspects of ourselves, to finally understand there is nothing that is not GOD, the ALL, and ALL of it is an expression of Divine Love. By integrating this knowledge into the wholeness that we are, we are finally free to express and explore our Self-Realization and Divine Expression.

The Heart: Connecting with Higher Vibrations

While we perceive the world as composed of solid objects, physics reminds us that at the atomic level, all matter is energy in motion. This understanding extends to our own bodies—our thoughts, emotions, and beliefs all generate energy fields that interact with the world around us.

Our heart is the most powerful electromagnetic source in the human body. Its electrical field is approximately 60 times greater in amplitude than that of the brain, and its magnetic field can be detected several feet away. This means that our hearts are like miniature satellites that send and receive energy waves and can detect unconscious energy fields, making it a potent force for transformation.

Modern science has proven that different emotions correspond to different vibrations. Our hearts emanate the frequencies corresponding to the vibration of our feelings, beliefs, emotions and mindset. These frequencies are like unseen radio waves—and we unconsciously attract people and circumstances that are aligned with the frequencies of our vibrations.

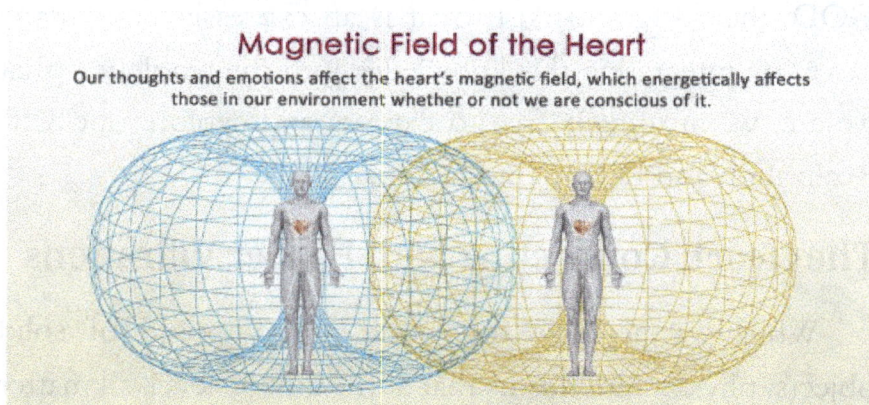

Magnetic Field of the Heart

Our thoughts and emotions affect the heart's magnetic field, which energetically affects those in our environment whether or not we are conscious of it.

Because our vibrational state influences what we attract into our lives, one of the keys to attracting what we desire is to raise our vibration, and the fastest way to raise our vibration is in our heart center.

But what does it mean to raise our vibration? It means to shift our focus and feelings from the lower wavelengths of shame, fear, blame or anger for example, into the higher wavelengths or vibrations of acceptance, courage, responsibility, and gratitude. When we shift our focus from the lower emotions on the vibrational scale and expand our hearts to vibrate with love, willingness, or gratitude, we align more closely with our Divine Nature.

Map of Consciousness Continuum

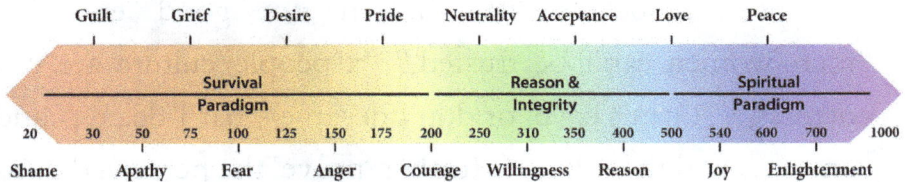

	Guilt		Grief		Desire		Pride		Neutrality	Acceptance		Love		Peace	

| | | | Survival Paradigm | | | | | | Reason & Integrity | | | | Spiritual Paradigm | | |

20	30	50	75	100	125	150	175	200	250	310	350	400	500	540	600	700	1000

| Shame | | Apathy | | Fear | | Anger | | Courage | | Willingness | | Reason | | Joy | | Enlightenment | |

Awakening The Heart to The Truth of Who We Are

Heart-Centered Healing Meditation is a modality that facilitates raising our vibration, healing past traumas, and observing where we are holding aspects of the ALL in separation. Through this process, we can make a conscious choice to integrate them into the Oneness through the love in our hearts. This process of energetic integration allows us to reclaim lost aspects of ourselves and to reconnect with the parts of ourselves that have been fragmented due to past pain, conditioning, or trauma. Through this process, we regain greater wholeness, peace, abundance and joy.

Let's break it down to clarify how this works...

Our heart center can feel blocked or be in a state of distrust, usually caused by painful childhood experiences or challenges. These incidents predispose us to protect ourselves from being vulnerable to anything resembling the original pain—even when we have grown, matured, and 'overcome' the original pain. However, that pain, even if we don't remember the occurrence that caused it, embedded in our subconscious beliefs like "I am not good enough," "men/women can't be trusted," "x people/culture are our enemies," "I can't have/or don't deserve what I desire," and son on... and these beliefs further 'prove' the perceived need for fragmentation and illusion of separation. It is as if a piece of us, our trust, our openness, our love, has stayed trapped in time when the incident occurred, and that unconscious part of ourselves keeps being triggered by life events or reacting as if we were still that child.

In the Heart Centered Healing Meditation Modality, we call these fragmented unconscious parts "Inner Children" who have stayed in separation from our True Self. These inner children have forgotten that they are a part of the ALL, a part of the Infinite expressions of GOD. However, the law of the Oneness reminds us that everything in creation is part of the ALL whether it is manifesting in the light or in the shadow.

The challenge is to remember that everything we experience and everything we are confronted with is all Divine Expression in its infinite possibilities, and that its purpose is always to lead us back to the love, the clarity, the Oneness that we are through the awakening of the heart.

When we start opening our heart back to the truth of who we are, acknowledging the parts of us we have held in separation, and start integrating these parts back through our heart by acknowledging the love they are, tremendous shifts and transformational healing occurs.

Healing Through Heart-Centered Awareness

Just as we carry within us "Inner Children," or wounded aspects of self that became trapped in time due to painful experiences, we may also harbor "Inner Male" or "Inner Female" energies that are in separation from our true essence. Through intentional heart-centered meditations we can heal these aspects by bringing them back into the embrace of Divine Love.

We do this by first acknowledging their presence and offering them compassion, understanding this is an aspect of ourselves and that we are bringing into Oneness with our hearts for our own wholeness. As you fill your heart with light and expand it to encompass all of the Oneness that you can, ask in your heart center:

'Am I willing to allow this Inner Child, Inner Female, or Inner Male to reveal the Truth that they are? Am I willing to receive them as Love?

Am I willing to surrender the illusion of separation that they are holding for me so that I can bring them back into the Oneness?'

Every aspect of life—or other humans—that we reject as a manifestation from Source, or a part of the ALL, is a mirror of the belief of separation we are holding and an invitation for us to transmute that belief. We don't have to like every aspect, person, or circumstance, but this process asks us to transform our beliefs and relationship with the energy we are holding about it, so that we can consciously receive them into wholeness out of love for ourselves.

Through our heart, we can transmute any belief, or any negative emotion, with compassion and the courage to Love ourselves more as ALL that we are. In doing so, we reclaim our full power and align ourselves with the universal flow of love and abundance.

Transformation Through Challenge

Humans are creatures of habit and when life is comfortable and going smoothly, we are rarely inspired to learn new ways of doing things or to search for personal growth. Pain, trauma, and challenges are usually life's greatest teachers. These are the catalysts that catapult us into looking for new perspectives, personal growth, healing and transformation—albeit sometimes kicking and screaming.

However, there is no need to wait for the body to get ill, or for a relationship to fall apart, or for a mid-life crisis to do the work that can magnify your wellbeing—and transform your life. Conscious, intentional healing is the most loving choice you can make to address any old wounds and challenges NOW. It is a choice to love yourself more.

By practicing the principles in this chapter and the Heart Center Healing Meditation (you will find a step-by-step guide at the end of the chapter), not only can you heal your mind, body and spirit, but you can often experience greater fulfillment in every aspect of your life.

Whatever challenges you may have had, or may be experiencing now or in the future, these practices can support you in your process.

➢ Heart Center Healing Meditation.

➢ Journaling, coaching, and energy work.

➢ Daily affirmations that help shift your mindset.

➢ Write down 3 things you can be grateful for every day (if you ever feel so down that you can't think of any, start with indoor plumbing and supermarkets).

➢ Acknowledge how small, daily choices (perspective shifts, habits, practices) contribute to your emotional recovery.

Understanding the Universal Laws provides a powerful framework for transforming our reality. The Law of Correspondence reminds us that our outer world is a reflection of our inner world. This means that how others treat us and the opportunities we attract reflect beliefs and emotions we are carrying inside. While the Law of Transmutation affirms that energy is always shifting and evolving, and we have the power to transmute our energy. By aligning our thoughts, beliefs, and emotions with Love and Gratitude, we become Conscious Creators of our reality.

When we feel disconnected, lost, or in pain, the key is not to resist these experiences but to use them as opportunities for deeper awareness. These are the moments we most need to tune into our hearts and practice these principles and daily tools. Every challenge presents us with an invitation to return to the truth of who we are. As we learn to attune ourselves to the wisdom of the heart, we become capable of transmuting lower vibrations and embodying the higher frequencies of love, gratitude, and unity.

The Heart: A Gateway to the Divine

The more we practice healing past events, pain, beliefs, and inner children, males, or females, the easier it becomes to trust our Heart Center and expand more into the Oneness. The more we connect with the vibration of Oneness, the more Love and Gratitude we experience. This becomes a circular exponential effect that leads us to greater peace, greater connection, and greater ability to attract what we desire.

As we grow with the practice of this meditation, we gain a greater understanding of our connection to ALL that is. We begin to see how everything that happens to us has a higher purpose. We experience a greater connection to all creation, from plants, animals, and humans to seeing the beauty of nature and perfection of the cosmos.

Our heart then becomes the center of our intuition, guidance, and knowingness. Through our heart we can tune in to our greater Divine Wisdom—our Higher Self—and when we do, we begin to experience all kinds of miracles.

Moving Forward with Intention & The Practice of Remembering

In the Heart-Centered Healing Meditation Guide, you are invited to work directly with these principles to release old wounds, integrate fragmented aspects of self, and elevate your vibration.

When you practice this meditation, simply notice what arises in your awareness—old memories, emotions, or patterns that may be calling for healing. Trust that everything is unfolding in Divine Timing and that you are experiencing exactly what you need to for your soul's evolution.

By embracing all aspects of yourself with love and compassion, you step into the fullness of your Divine Nature. You remember that you are, and always have been, part of the Infinite Oneness…

HEART CENTERED HEALING

MEDITATION GUIDE

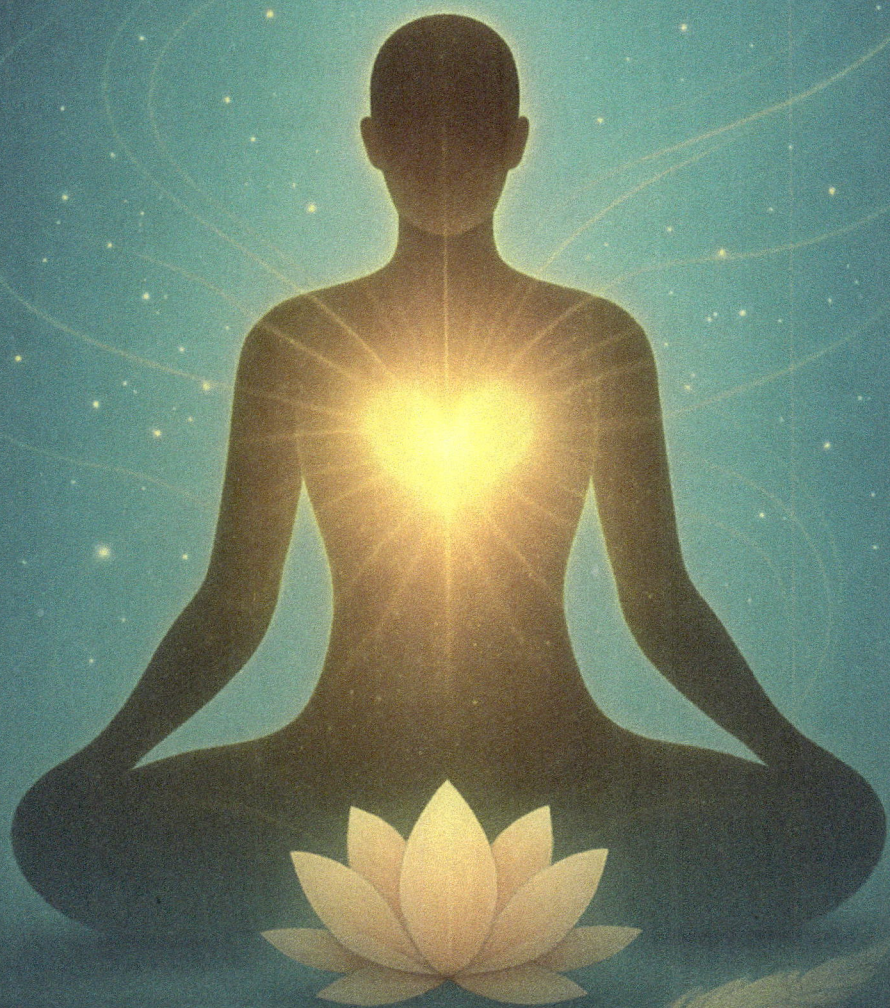

By Claudia Rocafort

Heart Centered Healing Meditation Guide

This Heart Centered Healing Meditation is designed to guide you back into alignment with your true essence—the Oneness of all that is. As you engage with this process, be willing to release any blocks or illusions of separation and embrace the Divine Love within and around you.

Read this guide through at least once before doing the meditation. I highly recommend recording the steps for yourself so that you can play them back and listen to them while you go through the meditation process. You can also go to my YouTube channel @ClaudiaRocafortCoaching or my website www.ClaudiaRocafortCoaching.com to access a complimentary recording of this guided meditation.

Scan for YouTube	Scan for Website

Now we will begin to connect, tune in, awaken, and expand your heart center. As you settle down comfortably in a chair, rest both palms on your legs, facing up to receive. Set your intention for your meditation by saying to yourself: "My heart is open to receive all the love that I AM. I am willing to receive and clear all that is for my highest purpose. Love flows through me and connects me to the Oneness that I AM."

Step 1: Find a Comfortable Position

Close your eyes and take a deep breath through your nose, filling your lungs fully. Slowly exhale through pursed lips as if you were blowing a candle gently, releasing with your breath any tension in your body. Allow your breath to become a calming rhythm, bringing you deeper into relaxation. With each exhale, feel your body sinking into a deeper state of peace.

Step 2: Feet on the Ground (preferably barefoot)

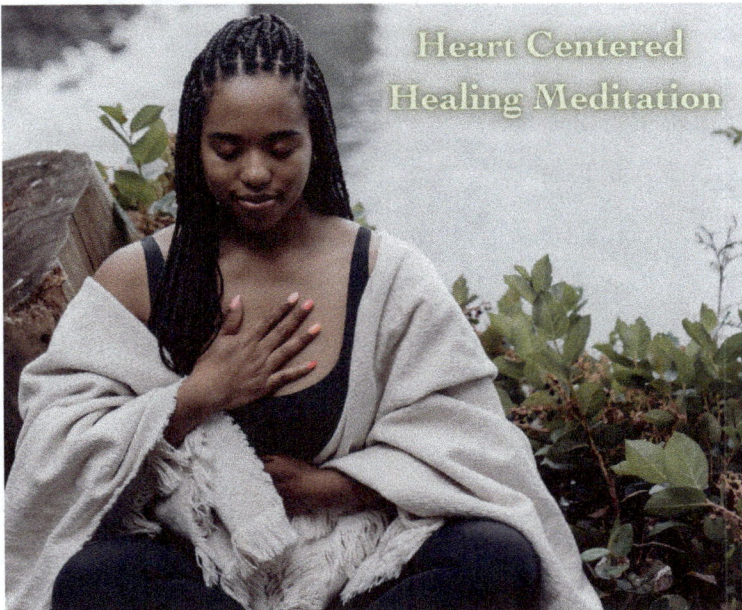

Heart Centered
Healing Meditation

Place your feet on the ground and feel the Earth's energy beneath you. Visualize roots growing from your feet, anchoring deep into the heart of the planet, providing you with stability, nourishment, and a deep connection to the natural world.

Step 3: Visualizing Golden Light in the Heart

Now, visualize a soft, warm, golden white light at the center of your heart. This radiant light represents the core of your being. Feel it expanding from your heart, gently nurturing every cell in your body with warmth and love. Let the energy of this light travel through your arms, down your legs, caressing every organ in your body, expanding up your spine, and to your crown, filling you with peace and a profound sense of connection to the Divine Love that you are.

Step 4: Expanding Beyond Time and Space

Allow this light to expand beyond the boundaries of your physical body. Feel it extending through time and space, connecting you with the higher frequencies of Love, Peace, and Gratitude. With each breath, feel the connection to Infinite Source—immerse yourself in this higher vibration of unity and Divine Presence. Bask in this gentle and powerful energy.

Step 5: Heart Center Connection

At the center of your being, feel yourself fully connected to the Oneness of the Universe and the Infinite Love of your Higher Self. Trust that your Heart Center holds the wisdom and healing energy you need. Allow any thoughts, feelings, or beliefs that arise to simply be—observe and acknowledge them as they arise.

Step 6: Asking for Guidance

In your Heart Center, ask Source, the Masters, Angels, and Guides: '*What am I meant to work on today? What am I meant to bring into the Oneness? What part of me is seeking healing or release?'* Allow the guidance to flow to you, trusting whatever arises is exactly what you are ready to embrace.

Step 7: Waiting for the Guidance

Allow yourself to gently wait and continue to expand the light and energy of your Heart. Trust that the right message will come to you. You may receive a vision, a memory, a sensation, or an inner knowing. You may remember a person or an event, feel a knowingness in your Heart, or hear an Inner Voice. You might become aware of a part of your body, feel some discomfort, or just get a sense that you are holding something in your body. Let the Guidance that arises flow through your heart into your awareness. There is no need to rush or force; simply trust in the Divine timing of this moment.

Step 8: Trusting the Process

Trust that Whatever arises it is exactly what you need most in this moment, that it is for your Highest Good, and that it is the perfect piece of your healing journey.

Step 9: Willingness to Transmute

Ask your Heart, *"Am I willing to transmute this in my heart and to let go of the illusion of separation? Am I willing to bring this into the Oneness that it is? Am I willing to receive this as the Love that it is?"*

Step 10: Working Through Resistance

If you experience any resistance, ask the part of you that is holding the resistance to reveal itself. You may become aware of an Inner Child, Inner Female or Inner Male. Allow them to show you what beliefs, feelings, pain, or separation they are holding.

Step 11: Working Through Emotions

If any emotions arise, allow them to flow gently through your Heart. Remember you are safe, and the emotions arising are meant to finally be acknowledged and released. Trust your heart to transmute any emotion, and to help you reveal the Love that it is.

Ask yourself *"Am I willing to see the Truth of this? Am I willing to receive this as Love? Am I willing to Love Myself more and allow this to be transmuted in my Heart? Am I willing to bring it back into the Oneness?"*

If you feel you need support, remember to Ask the Masters, your Angels, and Guides for their loving guidance and protection.

Step 12: Allow The Healing

Visualize the golden or white light in your Heart enveloping the feeling, person, event, Inner Child, Inner Female, or Inner Male that came up. Surround whatever has come up for you with the Infinite Love of Source and visualize IT becoming Light effortlessly.

Take your time and allow this process to unfold at its own pace. Visualize as everything that reveals itself integrates with the Light of the Oneness in your Heart.

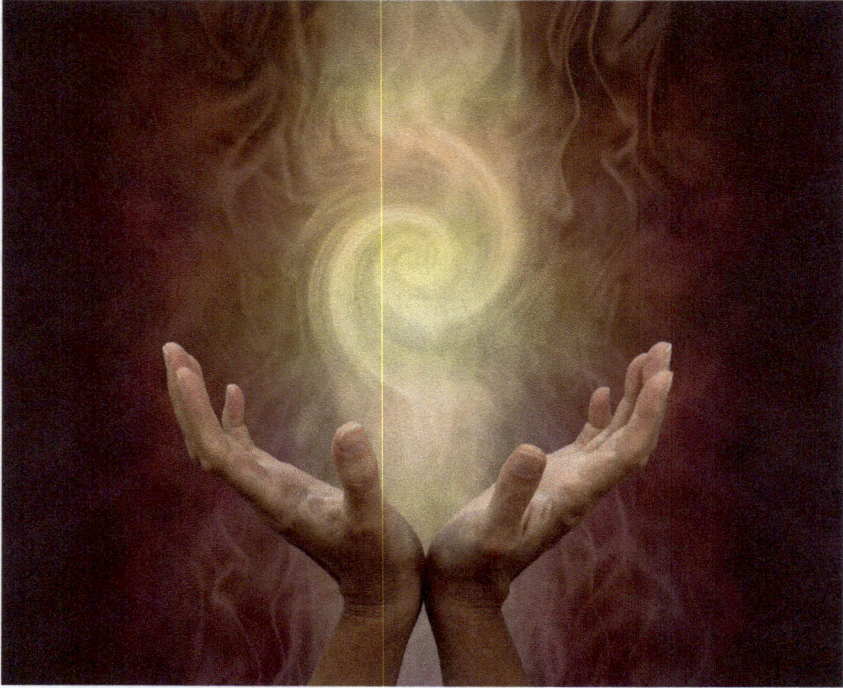

Step 13: Integration with The Oneness

As you expand your heart's light, know that you are not only healing yourself but contributing to the collective energy of Love and Oneness in the world. Each act of healing ripples outward, affecting all beings.

Notice how your heart feels lighter, more expansive, more connected to the Divine. As you allow everything to shift into Light and Love, let yourself bask in Gratitude for the healing taking place. Your light is now a beacon of love for all who are ready to receive it. Let this new feeling and energy infuse every part of you, knowing that this healing continues to unfold even after the meditation ends.

Step 14: Thank Source

When you feel guided to, set your intention in your heart for the process to continue to unfold through its integration, effortlessly. Thank the Masters, Angels, and Guides for their loving support. Thank your Heart, Source, God, or the Oneness for the Love and Healing received.

Step 15: Come Back to the Present Moment

Gently bring your awareness back to your body. Take a few deep breaths and feel your feet supported by the Earth beneath you. Slowly wiggle your toes, move your fingers, and gently stretch your body. Start bringing your awareness back into the room. When you feel ready, open your eyes, returning fully to the present moment. Set your intention to take the peace, wisdom, and connection from the Oneness with you throughout your day and close your session by saying "*Namaste*" ✦ ~ (The Divine Light in Me bows to the Divine Light in You)

After this type of work, always be very gentle with yourself. If possible, give yourself some time to rest and time to journal. Drink lots of water. Notice feelings and intuitions that arise. Follow any guidance you receive. You may experience new connections, and new awareness may come to you throughout the day. Acknowledge what you are grateful for from this experience.

I hope this chapter and guided meditation support your Highest Good and Highest Purpose. I look forward to holding space for you as you embark on this sacred journey back to the wholeness of your being. ✦

Please reach out to me if I can support you on your path. My holistic coaching approach incorporates mindset work, meditation and energy work, as well as the classic coaching tools and exercises that nurture well-being, cultivating peace, prosperity, and self-love. From clearing limiting beliefs to fostering conscious leadership, public speaking to strategic self-realization, my coaching empowers clients to step into their highest potential with clarity, confidence, and an open heart.

With Love & Light

Namaste ✦ **~ Claudia**

About the Author

Claudia Rocafort is an *alchemist of alignment*, seamlessly blending communication skills, mindset mastery, conscious leadership, meditation, and esoteric tools into coaching that transforms from the inside out.

A seasoned international actress turned ICF-certified coach, communication consultant, and spiritual facilitator, Claudia guides leaders and mission-driven achievers to unlock their zone of genius, clear limiting beliefs, and glow like pros—on stage, in business, or life.

Whether teaching public speaking and presentation skills, facilitating heart-centered healing meditations, or designing strategic action plans for self-realization and to level up your business.

Claudia's mission is clear: Lead with love. Communicate with clarity. Transform with truth.

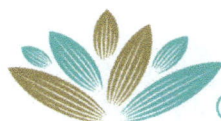

Claudia Rocafort Coaching
Create Conscious Conversations

Scan to contact Claudia

UNLOCKING SOUL-ALIGNED SUCCESS

RECLAIMING YOUR CLARITY, CONFIDENCE, AND CALM

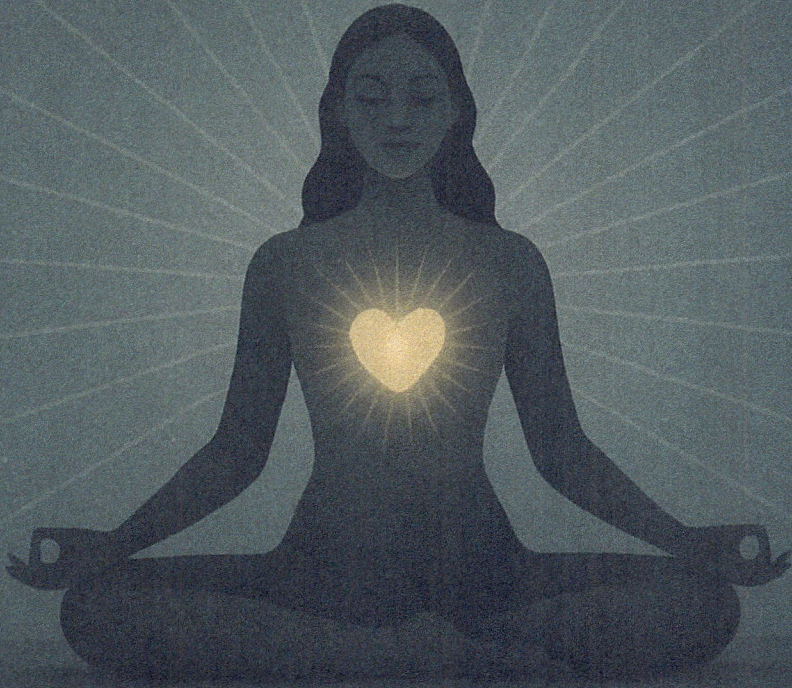

ANGELA NELSON

Clarity & Confidence Catalyst | *Hypnotherapist & Mindset Coach*

For my clients, past and present.
Your courage to heal inspires everything I do.

CHAPTER TWO

UNLOCKING SOUL-ALIGNED SUCCESS:

RECLAIMING YOUR CLARITY, CONFIDENCE, AND CALM

Angela Nelson, Clarity & Confidence Catalyst
| Hypnotherapist & Mindset Coach

"The wound is the place where the Light

enters you." - Rumi

Have you ever felt like you were living someone else's definition of success? Picture this: a high-performing professional woman, outwardly thriving yet inwardly struggling with an invisible battle that no amount of professional success could resolve. That was me, caught in the relentless cycle of striving for excellence while my body was quietly screaming for attention.

The Perfect Storm

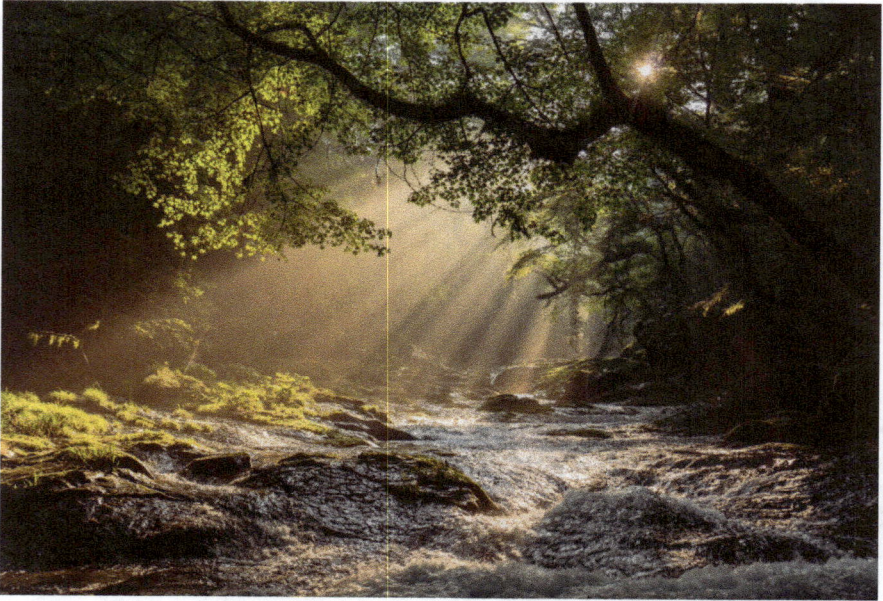

Dawn after dawn, I would wake to the familiar weight of exhaustion, my body a battlefield of autoimmune warfare. Psoriatic arthritis and rheumatoid arthritis weren't just medical diagnoses; they were unwanted companions that had infiltrated every aspect of my life. As someone who had built her identity around helping others and maintaining impossibly ambitious standards, the irony wasn't lost on me: I had become an expert at managing everything except my own wellbeing.

Like many of you, I was that person who could juggle multiple responsibilities with apparent ease. My calendar was a testament to efficiency, my achievements showed dedication, and my commitment to others was unwavering. Sound familiar? Yet beneath this carefully orchestrated exterior, chronic pain was rewriting my story, and relentless fatigue was dimming the light in my eyes.

Prior to my experience with chronic pain, I was a highly active and athletic individual. My schedule was full of various outdoor activities to counterbalance my work life, which was a high-pressure sales position with tradeshows and conventions- meaning a lot of hours on my feet and being quick on my feet. Don't get me wrong, I thrived in this environment and enjoyed meeting and working with people from all around the world. No day was ever the same and I enthusiastically embraced my work and the fast-paced environment.

My time away from work was spent volunteering in many capacities; as a Trail Crew Leader with the NPS (National Park Service), a Trip Leader with a local hiking club, a Ski Patroller with the NSP (National Ski Patrol), and doing river cleanups with a local riverkeeper. I hiked, kayaked, rock-climbed, and rappelled. The outdoors was my sanctuary, my love, and my life. That is, until the pain from previous traumas turned into chronic pain, and could no longer be ignored. My life began to unravel bit by bit as the pain spread throughout my body.

After years of pushing through the pain, my body began to succumb to the illnesses and I started losing my mobility, which took away what brought me the most joy- hiking and being outdoors. I was overcome with shame and tried my best to hide my condition from everyone. How could I explain what was happening to me when I didn't even understand it? I locked myself away, alone with my suffering. Aside from the multiple doctors' appointments that eventually took over my schedule, I rarely went out. The life I loved and embraced with all my heart and energy was taken away and all that was left was my broken body that became my painful prison. Little did I know that was only the beginning.

The onslaught of medications that followed and the many devastating side effects made my life close to unbearable. Pill after pill, I felt as if I was on a medicine merry-go-round, minus the merry, which wouldn't stop turning as it pummeled into a very dark abyss. Nothing worked to alleviate the extreme pain I was constantly burdened with, nor the sleepless nights due to the tormenting agony. My life had not only been turned completely upside down but had become a constant turmoil of torture. I wanted out.

The Breaking Point That Became My Breakthrough

The turning point came during another doctor's appointment. "There is nothing else we can do for you." Those words, clinical, final, devastating, hung in the air like a heavy fog. I drove home through the tears and collapsed on the floor. "Nothing else…?" "Get a wheelchair." "File for disability." The weight of those words came crashing down on me and I was lost in a sea of fear, hopelessness, and emptiness. But sometimes, when conventional wisdom reaches its limits, we're forced to look beyond the obvious.

In that moment of profound vulnerability, I did something I hadn't done in years: I became still. In the quiet space between despair and determination, I asked for guidance. I prayed like I had never prayed before asking God if he wanted me to live then to save me and then show me why he wanted me to be here. In that moment of stillness, I received clear divine guidance that would change everything, a powerful message that led me to discover the healing potential of holistic wellness.

"Let they food be they medicine…" The last thing I wanted to hear was the word 'medicine," but "How does food factor into this," I asked myself. Somehow, I made my way from the floor to the kitchen island where my laptop was. With my one, still functioning, crooked finger I began my search for what foods could help with the multitude of ailments that were wreaking havoc on my body.

The Body's Wisdom

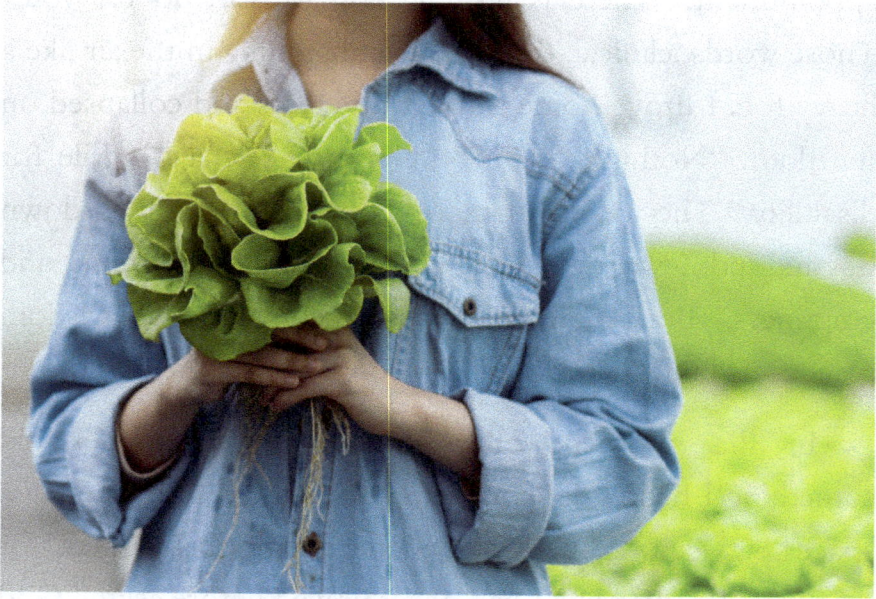

The first pillar of my transformation began with nutrition, not as a quick fix, but as a fundamental reconstructing of my relationship with food. My nutritional journey wasn't just about eliminating inflammatory foods, it was about discovering what truly nourished me at a cellular level. I learned that transformation happens in layers: first, removing what doesn't serve us, then rebuilding with nutrients that fuel vitality. For me, this meant discovering that certain "healthy" foods were actually contributing to my inflammation, while others I'd overlooked became powerful allies in my healing.

Through extensive research and experimentation, I discovered the transformative power of plant-based nutrition and whole food concentrations that could provide the comprehensive nutritional support my body had been craving.

The true nourishment went beyond supplementation. I embraced the profound connection between growing our own food and healing. Installing a vertical aeroponic garden system was more than just a source of fresh produce; it became a daily reminder of resilience and the power of nurturing, offering lessons that paralleled my own healing journey.

This foundation of physical nourishment laid the groundwork for the deeper mental and emotional healing achieved through introspection, reflection, and small mindset shifts.

I discovered the profound interconnectedness of mind, body, and spirit. The lessons I learned through this journey now form the foundation of my work as a Hypnotherapist & Mindset Coach. Read on to learn more about how these three areas of our being work together and how you can harness this power to lead a healthier and happier life.

The Mind's Power: Transforming from Within

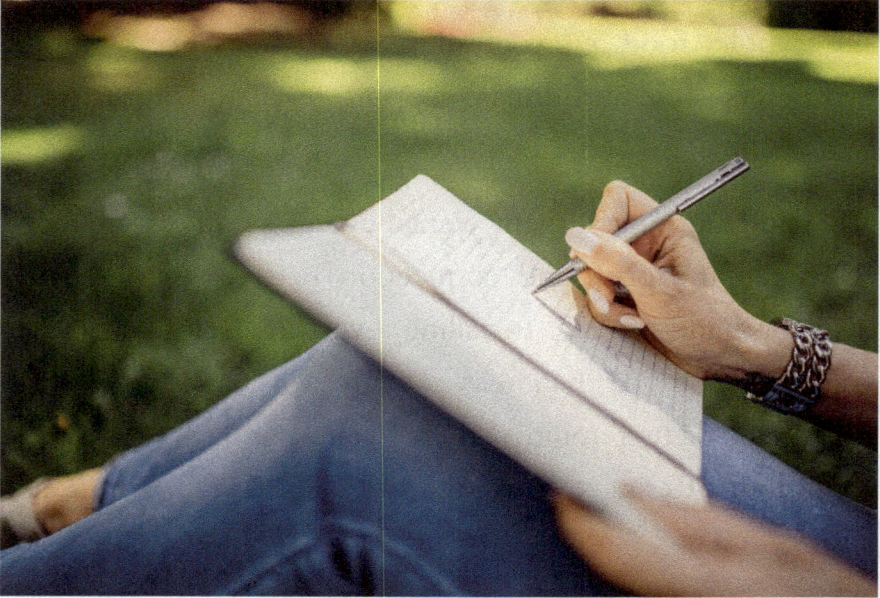

As I deepened my healing journey, I discovered two transformative approaches that would change not only my life but the lives of countless creative high performers I'd later work with: strategic mindset coaching and transformational hypnotherapy. These evidence-based modalities revealed a profound truth: our bodies often manifest what our minds cannot process.

While mindset work provides actionable tools for immediate change, hypnotherapy addresses the subconscious roots of emotional depletion and inner resistance. Together, these approaches create a powerful pathway to sustainable well-being and success. Through mindset discovery, I learned to identify and transform the thought patterns and beliefs that were programming my cellular response to stress. Hypnotherapy provided the key to accessing and rewiring these patterns at their source - the subconscious mind.

The results were revelatory: Those sleepless nights? They weren't only about physical pain; they were about unacknowledged trauma. The persistent fatigue? It wasn't just inflammation, it was years of saying "yes" when my soul was screaming "no." Hypnotherapy provided the clarity and release I needed to realign with my authentic self.

Today, I witness similar transformations in my clients. We uncover and heal the root causes of exhaustion, often tied to deeper patterns developed early in life. The outcomes are consistent and profound: clients resolve chronic insomnia, regain confidence, and implement wellness changes that ripple across their personal and professional lives. Many report sleeping through the night for the first time in years, achieving breakthroughs in work-life flow, and leading with renewed confidence.

These aren't isolated successes, they reflect the consistent impact of addressing both conscious patterns through mindset coaching and subconscious patterns through hypnotherapy. Together, these tools empower my clients to rebuild their lives with clarity, confidence, and calm. As clients rediscover their energy and clarity, their transformations extend beyond themselves, inspiring healthier habits among loved ones and fostering a culture of well-being within their families, teams, and organizations.

Consider one of my clients, an entrepreneur running a successful business yet constantly battling exhaustion. She poured all her energy into growing her company, believing that working harder was the only path to greater success. But behind the scenes, she was barely keeping up, sacrificing sleep, personal time, and even her health just to maintain the pace.

Through the combination of gentle mindset coaching and transformational hypnotherapy, she learned to shift her approach. She redefined what success meant beyond just revenue and milestones, set firm boundaries, and created sustainable habits that prioritized both her business growth and her well-being. Within months, she transitioned from barely staying afloat to leading her company with strategic clarity, grounded confidence, and a sense of calm she hadn't felt in years. She later told me, "I feel like I finally got my life back, but it's a life I've consciously chosen this time."

The Spirit's Journey

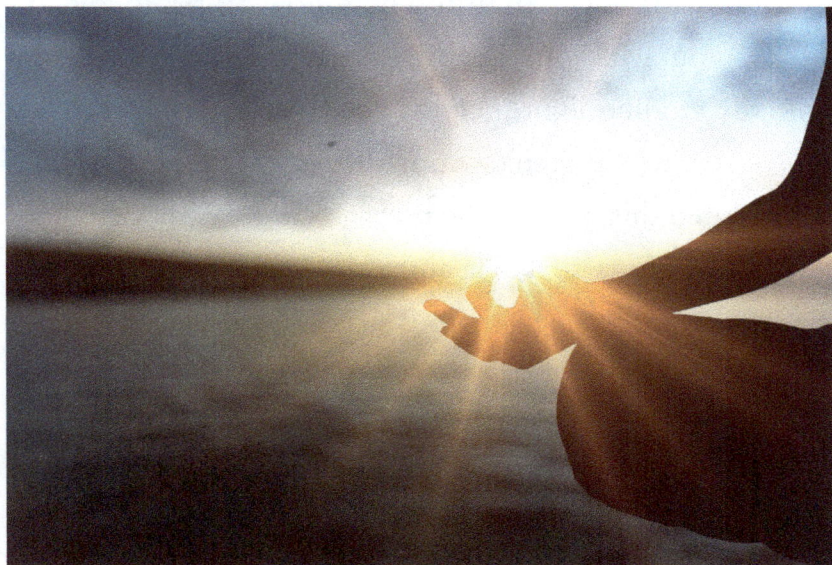

While mindset work and hypnotherapy address the mental and emotional aspects of transformation, my journey revealed another crucial dimension: spirituality. This aspect introduced me to faith and intuition as powerful tools for aligning with true purpose and navigating life's challenges with clarity.

The most profound aspect of my healing journey was the spiritual awakening. It initiated a deepening of my faith and a powerful recognition of the divine wisdom that guides us toward our highest purpose. Through daily prayer, meditation, journaling, and intentional silence, I began to hear the quiet voice of intuition that had been drowned out by the noise of constant doing.

This spiritual dimension taught me that true wellness transcends managing symptoms or following protocols, it's about aligning with our deepest truth and purpose. Faith became my guiding light, helping me trust the process even when outcomes weren't immediately visible. Intuition complemented this by allowing me to recognize opportunities and make decisions that felt authentic and aligned with my values.

Today, I integrate this spiritual perspective into my work with clients, enriching mindset coaching and hypnotherapy with practices that encourage connection with inner wisdom. For instance, a client struggling with career decisions learned to trust her instincts through guided meditations, leading her to opportunities that aligned with both her professional goals and personal fulfillment. Another client used hypnotherapy to uncover and transform deeply held fears that were blocking her from embracing her purpose.

Faith and intuition aren't separate from practical strategies, they amplify them. Together, they provide a holistic framework for transformation, ensuring that the journey is not only effective but deeply meaningful. Many clients report that reconnecting with their inner wisdom not only restores their energy and clarity but also reignites their sense of purpose and possibility.

The Birth of a Mission

As my own healing progressed, I felt called to expand my impact. This calling led me to pursue specialized training and certification in the most powerful modalities I had encountered on my own journey.

Today, I offer two powerfully complementary approaches to transformation:

High-Performance Mindset Coaching: A personalized approach to identifying and gently transforming limiting patterns, especially meaningful for mission-driven high performers who crave both results and inner alignment.

Transformational Hypnotherapy: A science-backed method for creating rapid, lasting change by accessing and reprogramming subconscious patterns.

These modalities work together to create comprehensive transformation, addressing both conscious strategies and subconscious programming.

I work with remarkable clients who appear to have it all together but inwardly feel a quiet disconnection from their essence. They come to me with symptoms that sound physical but often stem from deeper patterns:

The visionary creative who built a thriving brand, but quietly feels disconnected from the very purpose that once fueled her.

The certified coach who guides others with clarity but secretly questions her own path.

The soulful consultant whose body keeps sending signals, but who's afraid to slow down in case everything unravels.

Understanding the Deeper Patterns

Through my work with many high-performing professionals, I've identified three common patterns that contribute to mental depletion and persistent health challenges: The Achievement Trap, The Responsibility Paradox, and The Perfection Prison.

The Achievement Trap: When Success Feels Like a Moving Target

For high performers, success is often defined by achievement, recognition, and external validation. The thrill of accomplishment becomes addictive- closing the next deal, launching the next project, reaching the next milestone. Yet, with each success, the goalpost moves. There's no moment of arrival, only an endless chase.

This cycle is reinforced early. Many high-performing individuals grew up receiving praise for being smart, talented, or hardworking, which shaped their identity around proving their worth through doing. They learned that being "good enough" wasn't enough, they had to be the best.

The problem? Achievement alone doesn't create fulfillment. Many professionals reach impressive career heights yet still feel empty, restless, or dissatisfied. One coach I worked with realized she filled her calendar with back-to-back client calls and busy work, not because they were necessary, but because they validated her sense of importance. She was constantly holding space for everyone but herself.

To escape the Achievement Trap, we must redefine success. Sustainable success is not about constantly doing more; it's about aligning accomplishments with fulfillment and well-being. One transformative exercise is to ask: "If I could no longer measure my success by achievement, how would I define it?" For many proficient professionals, this question shifts their perspective from external validation to internal fulfillment. Instead of chasing more, they begin to focus on what truly matters, and sometimes that means doing less.

The Responsibility Paradox: When Taking Care of Others Means Neglecting Yourself

High performers are experts in responsibility. They are the ones people depend on, the ones who step up when things get tough, and the ones who carry the weight of businesses, teams, and even families on their shoulders. While responsibility is a strength, unchecked responsibility leads to mental and physical overload. Many take on more than they need to, not because they have to, but because they feel they should. The underlying belief? "If I don't do it, no one else will."

I see this often in creative high performers who feel the need to control every outcome, make every decision, and be the problem-solver for everyone around them. A business owner I worked with once shared, "I can't step away because everything depends on me." But the more she held onto everything, the more she found herself exhausted, overwhelmed, and disconnected from the bigger vision she had for her company. She knew she couldn't keep pushing like this, but didn't know how to slow down without losing momentum.

To release the Responsibility Paradox, high-achieving professionals must shift from over-responsibility to empowered leadership. They must recognize that leading does not mean doing everything, it means creating the right environment for success. A practical mindset shift is: "Who can I train, delegate to, or empower so I am not the bottleneck?" One of the most powerful transformations my clients experience is realizing that when they take care of themselves, they show up stronger for others.

The Perfection Prison: When Excellence Becomes a Barrier

For many high performers, perfectionism is a double-edged sword. It drives them to set ambitious standards, deliver exceptional results, and push beyond limits. But it also creates paralysis, self-doubt, and exhaustion.

Perfectionism often starts as a protective mechanism. It's the belief that if everything is perfect, I'll be safe, respected, or successful. However, in reality, perfectionism is fear disguised as excellence, fear of failure, fear of judgment, fear of not being enough.

One coach I worked with delayed launching her new program for months, obsessing over every detail. When we dug deeper, we discovered that her perfectionism was rooted in a fear of being criticized. She wasn't improving her work; she was avoiding visibility out of fear of being judged.

The antidote to the Perfection Prison is learning to embrace progress over perfection. Successful people thrive when they reframe failure as feedback and recognize that action beats endless preparation. A simple but powerful mindset shift is: "Done is better than perfect." Once my client embraced this, she launched her program within two weeks. Not only did it succeed, but she finally realized what her clients had needed all along, her grounded presence, not her perfection.

Final Thoughts: Why These Patterns Matter for High Performers

These three patterns, the Achievement Trap, the Responsibility Paradox, and the Perfection Prison, are not just concepts. They are the quiet, inherited patterns shaping how many high performers think, feel, and respond. Left unexamined, they lead to chronic stress, emotional fatigue, and quiet dissatisfaction. But once recognized, they become the key to transformation. For high performers who are done with surface-level work and ready for deeper healing, recognizing these patterns is the first step to reclaiming their clarity, confidence, and calm.

By shifting from achievement addiction to fulfillment, from over-responsibility to empowered leadership, and from perfectionism to progress, high performers can reclaim their clarity, confidence, and calm, while creating sustainable success.

Which of these patterns do you resonate with most?

A Framework for Transformation

Drawing from my personal journey and professional expertise, I developed a transformative experience that addresses the unique challenges faced by high-performing professionals. What makes my approach truly distinctive is the deeply personalized attention I bring to each client. I understand the unique challenges high-performing professionals face and tailor strategies to meet their individual needs.

Leading with my heart and driven by a passion for transformation, I guide my clients to become the healthiest, happiest versions of themselves, fostering not just success but genuine fulfillment.

This isn't another "quick fix" program; it's a comprehensive approach that balances your professional demands with your personal well-being. Through the strategic combination of mindset shifts and hypnotherapy, we create lasting transformation. Each session is tailored to your unique needs and goals, ensuring your journey to wellness integrates seamlessly into your life. My clients consistently report profound results- renewed clarity, confidence, and a calm sense of direction, while achieving even greater professional success.

The ripple effect of transformation is truly inspiring. When professionals reclaim their vitality and clarity, they empower not only themselves but also their teams, practices, and organizations. This shift from depletion to vitality fosters resilience, promotes calm focus, and drives sustainable productivity. It creates a lasting legacy of wellness, cultivating a culture of well-being and collaboration that extends far beyond individual success.

If you're craving more than surface-level fixes and want real, lasting change that honors your mind, body, and spirit, this work was created for you.

Your Path to Transformation

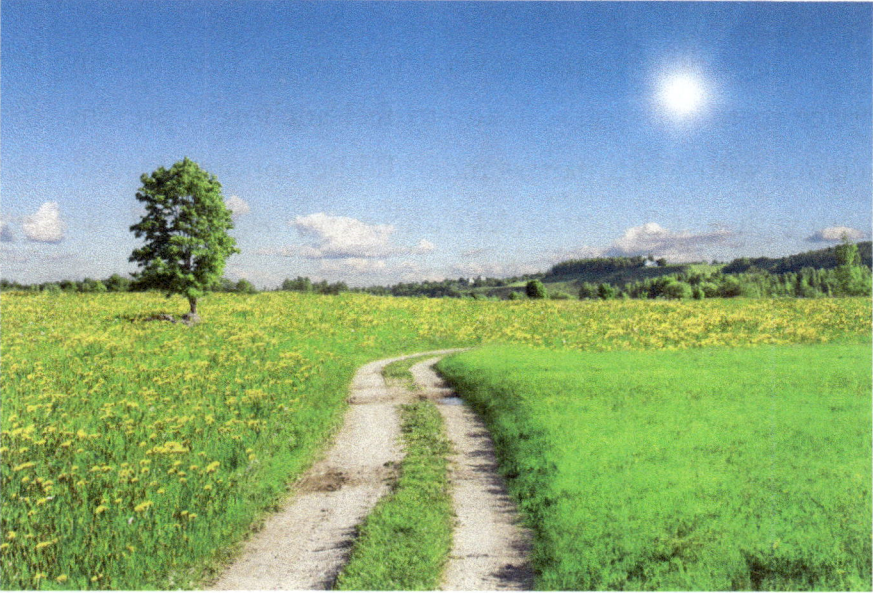

If you're ready to shift from exhaustion to sustainable success, let's explore what that looks like for you when you schedule a Complimentary Connection Call by visiting my website. Together, we'll uncover your challenges and design a personalized path forward. With sessions conducted entirely online, clients can prioritize transformation from anywhere, seamlessly fitting into their demanding schedules.

Looking back at my journey, from chronic illness to vibrant health, from overextension and emotional depletion to a life of purpose and alignment, I'm filled with deep gratitude. Not only for the healing I experienced, but for the sacred opportunity to guide others back to their own clarity, confidence, and calm.

Your brilliance has never left you; it's been waiting for space to rise. If you're ready to feel anchored, present, and aligned with what matters most, I'd be honored to walk that path with you. Together, let's uncover what's already within.

Let's Connect

Let's connect and take the first step toward reclaiming your clarity, confidence, calm, and sustainable success.

CoachAngelaNelson.com

Angela Nelson is the Clarity & Confidence Catalyst | Certified Hypnotherapist & Mindset Coach who helps high-performers unlock clarity, confidence, and calm by releasing the subconscious patterns quietly holding them back.

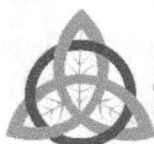

About the Author

Angela Nelson is a Clarity & Confidence Catalyst | Certified Hypnotherapist & Mindset Coach who helps high performers unlock clarity, confidence, and calm by releasing the subconscious patterns quietly holding them back.

After overcoming her own journey through autoimmune illness and perfectionism-fueled depletion, Angela discovered the profound link between subconscious mastery, emotional clarity, and soul-aligned success.

Today, she works with coaches, consultants, and creative entrepreneurs who often feel mentally drained, quietly disconnected, or stuck behind the scenes of their own success. Through her signature process, Angela helps her clients reclaim clarity, confidence, and calm—so they can lead their lives and businesses with greater ease, purpose, and integrity.

Her approach blends practical mindset coaching with science-backed hypnotherapy to help clients stop overthinking, gently shift unconscious patterns, and step fully into the next chapter of their success—feeling grounded, energized, and aligned.

Learn more: CoachAngelaNelson.com
https://Angela.TowerGarden.com
https://Angela.JuicePlus.com

NEUROTRANSMITTERS
REVEALED

THE ART AND SCIENCE OF
HEALING BRAIN CHEMISTRY

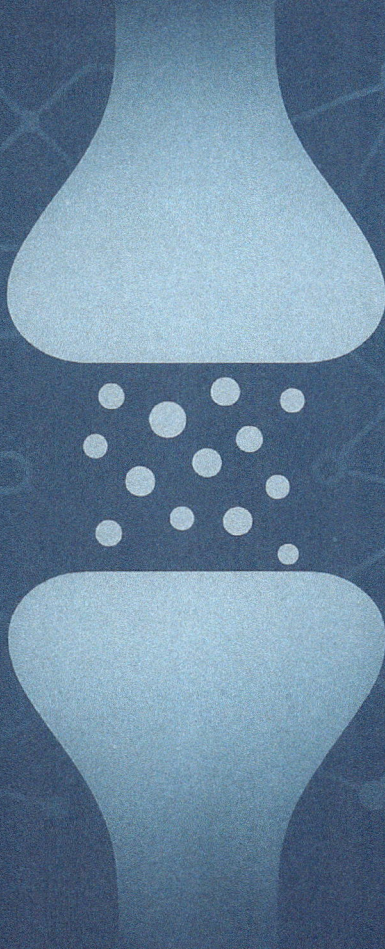

TAMARA OWEN, RN, MS, PMHNP

Chapter Three

Neurotransmitters Revealed:

The Art and Science of Healing Brain Chemistry

Tamara Owen, RN, MS, PMHNP

Have you ever thought about where your energy, motivation, focus, concentration, memory, and all the other mental and physical resources we rely on each day, actually come from? What about your mood, sleep, or appetite? I have to admit, I never really thought about it either. These things just seemed to exist, shifting seemingly randomly, sometimes causing problems, other times bringing moments of joy. But once I began to dig deeper and understand what regulates our emotions and drives our behavior, this knowledge transformed me, not only as a person but also in how I approach my work as a mental health nurse practitioner.

Before I started doing the work I do now, I was always intrigued by natural healing practices and the idea of treating conditions without medications or invasive procedures. While this approach seemed noble, it didn't always work out as I'd hoped. I spent a lot of time reading natural health articles, journals, and learning about supplements for various mental health conditions. I even tried taking some of them myself, despite there being little to no scientific evidence that they would actually help with my particular symptoms or concerns. Most of these supplements didn't seem make much of a difference, and I try not to think too hard about all the money I spent on them over the years.

Everything changed for me as a mental health nurse practitioner in 2006 when I first learned about brain chemistry, neurotransmitter testing, and treatment. That discovery unlocked an entirely new path for both exploration and healing. The art and science of balancing brain chemistry became, and remains, the most rewarding challenge in my practice. I soon realized that while therapy can be incredibly helpful, if your brain chemistry is out of balance, no amount of counseling will bring your mental health to the level you desire. It's like trying to build a house on an unstable foundation, no matter how much work you put in, the results just won't stick.

I've also come to understand a fundamental scientific truth that shapes our lives: we are chemical, electrical, and energetic beings. If our chemistry and electrical systems are out of balance, how can we expect to feel healthy, vibrant, and fully able to express ourselves as we're meant to? Without harmony in these core elements, it's nearly impossible to experience life with the energy and vitality we desire. This understanding drives me both personally and professionally, every single day.

Like most mental health practitioners, I have my own personal journey that has shaped both my life and my practice, leading me to become the person I am today.

I grew up in a chaotic household with five siblings, six horses, two dogs, and usually at least a cat or two. One year, we even hosted an exchange student, making us seven kids in a house that wasn't built for this many beings. It wasn't a mansion, nor was it in a spacious countryside setting, it was a modest home that my father kept adding onto in a constant effort to accommodate our growing family. As a result, we were cramped, shared rooms, and had no real privacy.

As the third child and a sensitive soul, I often felt like there was never any peace or quiet. From the moment I woke up, there was always work to do, daily chores, taking care of the animals, taking care of my siblings, until finally, after dinner, I'd sit down to do homework. Being a natural morning person, by then I had little energy or brainpower left for studying.

What really affected me, though, was the constant fighting. Whether it was with my older sister, younger brother, or my mother, or my brothers fighting amongst themselves, there always seemed to be tension and anger in the house. More than anything, it was the constant conflict and the harsh criticism from my mother that took a heavy toll on my mental health. I was no stranger to standing up for myself with my siblings, but when it came to my mother, I would shrink back, arguing with her only brought more distress, so I learned to avoid it.

I didn't realize the full extent of the emotional damage until I was an adult. It wasn't until my thirties, when I began to actively work on healing, that I recognized I'd been living with depression for most of my life. It was only after coming out of a particularly deep slump that I realized I felt better, and that's when it hit me: those lows had been depression all along. Over time, I started to experience more frequent mood swings, with the "highs" lasting longer and longer. Reflecting on my childhood and teenage years, I realized I had been living in a constant fog, always trying to escape the harsh reality of my chaotic home. I didn't fully grasp the lasting effect it would have on my adult life and relationships.

I struggled with intense anger issues, but having been taught from a young age that expressing my anger was unacceptable, I suppressed it. Instead, it would seep out in small doses, through snide or inappropriate comments and passive aggressiveness, that ultimately pushed away those closest to me. Instead of expressing my true feelings outwardly, my anger also turned inward and manifested as anxiety. While it was completely destructive to my body, anxiety felt more acceptable in public. Anger (Fight) and anxiety (Flight), both part of the stress response, are natural reactions designed to protect us from danger. They trigger a flood of chemicals in the body and brain, propelling us into action. This can be helpful if we're running from a lion and require a surge of adrenaline, but over time, these excess chemicals cause lasting damage, not just to our physical bodies, but to our mental health as well.

Throughout my childhood and into adulthood, anger and anxiety constantly alternated within me, and I battled daily headaches as a result. I often felt like a "bee in a bottle," frantic to escape the emotions I was desperately trying to keep a lid on. Much of my life was spent longing for that escape, as "sensitive me" was constantly on high alert, reacting to my mother's moods and the actions of others, when even the slightest thing someone else did or said would trigger memories of her. I often felt hurt by those around me, even though on some level, I knew their intentions weren't malicious. I was in awe of anyone who could just let things roll off their back, seemingly unaffected by words or actions.

My heightened sensitivity and reactivity began to take a toll on my relationships, not just with my mother, but with friends and family as well. I realized I needed to build a thicker skin and develop healthier coping skills. However, I couldn't simply force myself to stop being sensitive, and suppressing my reactions only intensified my internal anger and anxiety. The only advice I had ever received when I had intense reactions was to "snap out of it" or, as my grandfather used to tell me, "pull yourself up by your bootstraps and soldier on." I had never been taught any realistic coping or communication skills that I could actually implement in my relationships.

I had already done a lot of therapeutic work, talk therapy, somatic body work, and hypnotherapy. I knew that gaining better life skills would be beneficial, so I enrolled in countless courses to learn how to function better as an adult, especially in ways my family hadn't taught me. These included training in communication and relationship skills, conflict resolution, stress management, relaxation, and neurolinguistic programming. I attended lectures, read books, and devoured articles. But despite all these efforts, nothing seemed to cure me of my "bee in a bottle" frenzy, as I had come to think of it, or elevate my mood in a lasting, sustainable way.

During graduate school, I developed insomnia. I rarely saw doctors, but by this point I was desperate. Fortunately I was able to receive treatment from a compassionate physician at the University Student Health Center. She prescribed Trazodone to help me sleep, and it worked like a charm, along with the unexpected benefit of easing the irritability and anger I'd been carrying around since childhood. To me, it felt like a miracle. I was sleeping better, but I was still wound up, like a jack-in-the-box, as my doctor humorously demonstrated by winding the toy and then lifting her hands dramatically when "Jack" popped out. That vivid memory of her spot-on demonstration has always stayed with me, as it perfectly captured the anxiety I was feeling.

To address my lingering anxiety, my doctor prescribed Zoloft, an SSRI antidepressant that also helps with anxiety. At first, the idea of taking an antidepressant, something that seemed at odds with my preference for "natural" treatments, felt daunting and counterintuitive. But I trusted her judgment and deferred to her expertise. I had been suffering for so long, and honestly, my anxiety had worn me down.

Three months into taking Zoloft, I realized something remarkable: all the little things that used to trigger my anger, stress, and irritation had faded. Another miracle! What a relief it was to finally experience a level of peace after years of living with mental anguish. It was tempting to stay in that state, or assume that I would stay on the medication to feel this way, forever. But after eight months, I had a loud, unmistakable voice in my head that said simply: "Go off the Zoloft." There was no repetition, just a clear, direct intuition that I couldn't ignore. I felt as if it were the voice of God, or at least God not so subtly nudging my intuition, so certain and compelling that I knew I had no choice but to obey. So, I safely tapered off the medication.

Taking Zoloft for those eight months was nothing short of miraculous for me, as you've likely noticed from my repeated use of the word, but alas no other word comes close to describing the feeling. It elevated my life to a whole new level of meaning and fulfillment, where I no longer experienced anxiety or depression the way I once had. In fact, I haven't felt depressed since. I still experience moments of sadness, of course, but not depression. I also still feel anxious at times, especially when overwhelmed or juggling too much, but I'm no longer that frantic "bee in a bottle," that I once was, trapped in a cycle of mental chaos. I learned that when used judiciously, medications have an important role in health and healing.

To maintain my well-being and stay free from anxiety, depression, and other mental health challenges, I felt it would be beneficial to incorporate a non-pharmaceutical approach for ongoing support. My professional passion lies in helping others achieve vibrant health, and I realized I wanted the same lifestyle for myself. While I was healthy on paper, achieving true vibrancy requires more than just excellent self-care, it demands balance in all aspects of life, including the delicate harmony of our brain chemicals.

As chemical, electrical, and energetic beings, achieving true vibrant health requires addressing and healing all three aspects. While therapy and learning new skills can offer valuable support, an imbalance in our neurotransmitters can make life feel like an ongoing struggle, even when we're working hard to reach our goals.

Neurotransmitters, our brain's chemical messengers, play a critical role in regulating countless functions that shape our daily lives. When these are out of balance, we can experience discomfort, challenges in managing emotions, and difficulty functioning effectively.

Several factors can contribute to neurotransmitter imbalances, including:

➤ Stress in the physical, mental and emotional forms

➤ Poor diet or an inability to absorb and utilize nutrients from food

➤ Insufficient self-care, such as inadequate sleep, lack of exercise, and not taking time to relax and de-stress

➤ Infections

➤ Genetics

➢ Exposure to environmental toxins

➢ Substance abuse

➢ Organ dysfunction

➢ And more

Here's a short questionnaire to help you determine if balancing your neurotransmitters might be beneficial for you.

Do you experience any of the following symptoms or conditions? (Listed in no particular order):

Questionnaire: Could balancing your neurotransmitters help you?

Please answer Yes or No to the following questions:

1. Do you experience difficulty sleeping?

2. Do you have trouble losing or gaining weight?

3. Do you have low energy?

4. Do you often feel fatigued?

5. Do you experience low moods?

6. Do you struggle with poor concentration or trouble learning?

7. Do you experience moodiness?

8. Do you experience mood swings?

9. Do you have frequent aches and pains?

10. Have you noticed blood sugar changes that could lead to diabetes?

11. Do you get sick often (indicating a low immune system)?

12. Do you have intestinal complaints?

13. Do you feel anxious or experience anxiousness?

14. Do you struggle with social anxiety?

15. Do you have obsessive-compulsive tendencies or behaviors?

16. Do you hoard things or struggle to get rid of things?

17. Do you find it hard to cope with daily life stressors?

18. Do you often feel irritable?

19. Have you had angry outbursts?

20. Are you sensitive to certain triggers or situations?

21. Have you stopped enjoying things you once loved?

22. Do you experience PMS symptoms?

23. Are you dealing with menopause symptoms?

24. Do you experience urges and cravings?

25. Do you struggle with any kind of addiction?

26. Have you noticed a decrease in motivation?

27. Do you feel easily distracted?

28. Do you have poor focus or concentration?

29. Do you experience forgetfulness or poor memory?

30. Do you feel like you have "brain fog"?

31. Are you impulsive?

32. Do you have poor or sluggish cognition (thinking)?

33. Do you feel like you have excess energy?

34. Do you often ruminate (get stuck in repetitive thoughts)?

35. Does your mind race?

36. Do you have a hard time completing tasks?

If you answered "yes" to any of these symptoms or conditions, know that you are not alone. Many people are struggling needlessly, but here's the good news: you don't have to continue suffering.

My preferred approach to working with clients is to begin with solid data. The first test I rely on is a genetic test specifically designed for mental health. While this test is primarily used to guide medication choices, it also provides valuable insights into genes that may not be functioning optimally and how they might affect mental and emotional health.

The process is simple: a saliva sample is collected using Q-tips swabbed inside the cheek and sent to the testing lab. This test provides a basic understanding of how a client's brain chemistry system functions on a genetic level. It also offers insights into how the body processes medications, shedding light on the efficiency of genes responsible for breaking down medications.

Think of the "Goldilocks and the Three Bears" analogy:

Papa Bear's chair: Genes break down medication too quickly, leaving insufficient amounts in circulation.

Mama Bear's chair: Genes break down medication too slowly, leaving excess medication in the body.

Baby Bear's chair: Genes function correctly, breaking down medication at the right pace to ensure optimal levels in circulation.

Having this information helps in choosing medications that are most effective for each individual while minimizing side effects. It also eliminates guesswork by identifying medications that may not be as effective.

For those who prefer to avoid medications, knowing which genes are underperforming allows me to recommend supplements tailored to support those genes and promote balance naturally.

Another valuable test is a neurotransmitter test, which offers detailed insights into neurotransmitter biomarkers. Urine samples are collected throughout the day and sent to the testing lab for analysis. The results not only reveal neurotransmitter levels but also provide critical information about cortisol levels, which significantly impact our energy levels throughout the day. In my experience, clients' symptoms consistently align with these biomarkers. These tests are fascinating and provide essential data for creating a personalized treatment plan.

Targeted amino acid therapy can help bring neurotransmitters into better balance, while adaptogens, natural substances, often herbs or plant extracts, support the adrenal glands by enhancing the body's ability to resist stress and maintain homeostasis.

Amino acids, the building blocks of proteins, are fundamental for neurotransmitter production and regulation. A diet rich in amino acids is essential, with animal proteins being the most concentrated source. There are nine essential amino acids that the body cannot produce on its own, making it crucial to obtain them through diet. While supplementation is sometimes recommended, the goal is to meet these needs through proper nutrition.

Beyond the essential amino acids, the body can manufacture additional "non-essential" amino acids from these nine. Despite being termed "non-essential," these amino acids are equally vital for physical and mental health. However, factors like protein deficiency, poor nutrition, excess toxicity, or chronic stress can lead to deficiencies in these non-essential amino acids, impacting overall health and well-being.

Several factors can lead to suboptimal levels of amino acids, including:

➤ Lack of protein in the diet: This can result from either insufficient protein intake or a poorly balanced vegan/vegetarian diet.

➤ Poor digestion: Inefficient digestion can impair the absorption of amino acids from food.

➤ Genetic factors: Certain genetic predispositions can affect how well the body utilizes and processes amino acids.

➤ Toxicity: Exposure to toxins can interfere with the body's ability to properly synthesize and use amino acids.

> ➤ Latrogenic causes: These are side effects of medical treatments, such as medications, that can disrupt amino acid balance.

To sum up, amino acids are the essential building blocks of neurotransmitters, making them crucial for proper brain function and mental health. A diet rich in high-quality protein and essential nutrients is key to supporting optimal neurotransmitter production and promoting emotional and cognitive well-being. I work closely with my clients to educate them on the importance of diet in maintaining and balancing their neurotransmitters for overall health.

Here's how it all works together:

The balance of our brain chemistry, along with the function of our immune and endocrine (hormonal) systems, governs how we feel and function throughout our day. Our brain is the control center that dictates our physical, mental, and emotional states. The balance of amino acids is crucial in this process, as each neurotransmitter plays a specific role, often requiring collaboration between several. When these systems are out of balance or not working together as intended, we can experience a wide range of symptoms, as outlined in the questionnaire you answered above.

Balancing our neurotransmitters is not just about brain chemistry, it's about healing our whole body and practicing excellent self-care. This includes getting adequate sleep, exercising regularly, and eating nutritious foods. We also need time to rest and actively manage our stress. All of these factors contribute to neurotransmitter balance. To become our most vibrant selves, we must pay attention to and spend time improving all of these areas. Once our brain is healthier and more balanced, we feel calmer, more relaxed, and life begins to feel easier. This is when therapy and skill-building can truly take effect.

Deciding to get healthy from the inside out is like building your dream house, you wouldn't start choosing furniture and decor without first ensuring the foundation and structure were solid, right? Lay the foundation, build strong walls, install a reliable roof, and create a home that will support you for years to come.

I feel incredibly fortunate to have discovered neurotransmitter testing and treatment early in my career as a mental health nurse practitioner. In the mid-2000s, my doctor focused on healing from the inside out and introduced me to neurotransmitter testing and treatment. After taking the test, a simple urine collection, I began using the recommended supplements. It was a valuable experience to see how these supplements worked on my own body while learning the biochemistry from experts in the field. Not only did this approach work wonders for me, but it also freed me from relying on antidepressants ever again.

What I've learned about brain chemistry has been pivotal in shaping my practice. It has equipped me with the knowledge and tools to support my clients in a way that aligns with my values. Over the past 20 years, this has allowed me to help countless individuals achieve true health and vitality, safely, without the long-term side effects of pharmaceuticals. Additionally, I've built a strong network of naturopathic doctors with whom I collaborate to create holistic treatment plans that address the mind, body, and spirit.

Our world is moving at an ever-increasing pace, and it will continue to do so. How can we keep our minds and bodies in alignment and manage our stress effectively? Striving for balance is the key. Achieving this balance requires commitment, self-awareness, knowledge, and the willingness to make healthy choices every single day. The temptations and disruptors, both internal and external, will always be there, but knowing how to tune into our bodies and our

needs will guide us every step of the way. We're not striving for perfection, we're striving for consistent daily practice. Each day may look a little different, and that's okay. Some days, you'll power through your entire to-do list and still have energy to spare. Other days, you might need to curl up on the sofa with a good book, and both are equally valuable, as long as you're tuning in to what your body needs. Self-care is a lifelong journey with no days off, but the rewards are immeasurable.

My own journey continues to evolve as I learn more about what it truly takes to be healthy in mind, body, and spirit, and most importantly, what works well for my unique lifestyle. I, too, face the daily challenge of staying on the path of self-care and tuning into my body and its needs. With so many distractions and temptations in life, it's easy to veer off course. However, I'm grateful that I now understand what my brain and body need in terms of supplementation, and I no longer waste money on supplements or quick fixes that don't serve my long-term well-being. While I'm no longer that "bee in a bottle" girl I once was, I look back on her with fondness and gratitude, for all she taught me and for guiding me to where I am today.

There are many modalities that support health and healing included in this book. I always encourage my clients to explore different approaches, as there is no one-size-fits-all path, so I'm honored to be amongst so many talented practitioners with unique skillsets. Healing brain chemistry is a vital part of self-care, and working with someone who understands both the art and science of this process can be transformative. Balancing our brain chemistry requires education, guidance, and testing, and with the right approach, it's absolutely achievable. This can be just one aspect of your journey toward true healing and vibrant health for your mind, body and spirit.

If you're interested in healing your brain chemistry, I invite you to visit my website and sign up for a complimentary educational consultation. During this session, we can explore whether neurotransmitter testing, and follow-up care are a good fit for you.

Vibrant health,

Tamara

About the Author

Tamara Owen is a Psychiatric Mental Health Nurse Practitioner specializing in neurotransmitter testing and holistic mental health care. With over 25 years of experience, she has helped countless clients achieve lasting well-being through cutting-edge brain chemistry testing, targeted nutrition, and personalized treatment plans that support optimal health in mind, body, and spirit.

Her journey into this work began with both curiosity and frustration. Before discovering the science of brain chemistry, Tamara spent years exploring natural remedies and supplements with limited success. Everything changed when she learned how the brain's chemical messengers shape our thoughts, feelings, and behaviors. That knowledge transformed not only her own life but also the way she supports others in her work. Today, she blends the art and science of neurotransmitter testing and treatment in her practice, helping clients uncover the root causes of their symptoms and guiding them toward more vibrant, energized lives. Tamara's mission is to help women master their health and well-being so they can start living a more meaningful and passionate life. We are chemical, electrical, and energetic beings, and when those systems come into balance, everything begins to shift.

Want to go deeper? Download my free guide to see if balancing your brain chemistry is the right next step for you:

https://https://www.tamaraowen.com/neurotransmitter-guide

Website: https://tamaraowen.com

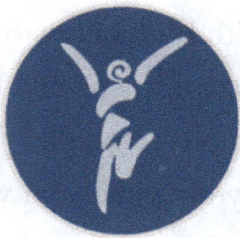

TAMARA
Owen
RN, MS, PMHNP

THE
SILENT SHIFT
NO ONE
WARNED US
ABOUT

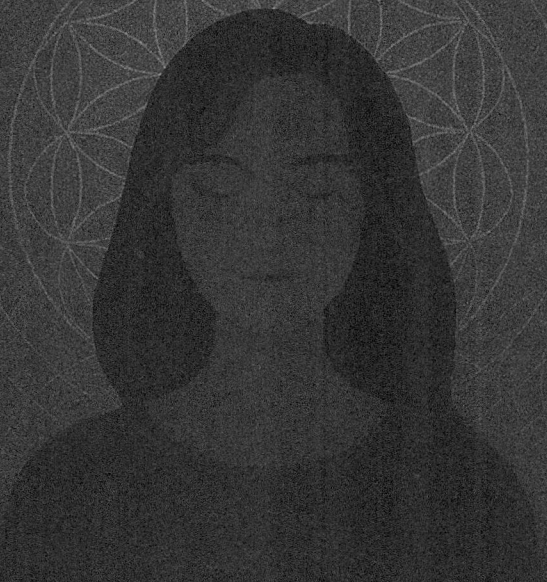

APRIL RANARD, CHLC

CHAPTER FOUR

THE SILENT SHIFT NO ONE WARNED US ABOUT

April Ranard, CHLC

You wake up one morning and something feels... different. It's not tiredness; it's exhaustion that wraps around your bones and sits heavy in your spirit. Your jeans don't fit, your brain is foggy, and your mood swings faster than you can keep up with. You wonder, *What is happening to me?*

The worst part? You feel like you're the only one going through it. Like no one warned you. No one prepared you.

But here's the truth: you are not alone. And you're not broken.

Perimenopause is a natural change that impacts many women. It affects their emotions, physical health, and spiritual well-being. It's the rollercoaster we never saw coming. It's a silent ride passed down from generations who lacked the tools to speak up. Our mothers and grandmothers suffered in silence. Today, we don't have to, and we can and should make a different choice. We can choose awareness, education, healing,

and community.

This is for women who feel lost in their bodies. If you're confused by symptoms you can't explain, you're not alone. It's okay to fear that this "new normal" might last forever. This is for the woman who looks in the mirror and doesn't recognize herself. It's for the woman whose spark feels dimmed.

This is for the woman who is ready to reclaim her power, her health, and her voice - who feels like it will never return.

What is Perimenopause?

Perimenopause refers to the years surrounding the time when you are transitioning to menopause. It can start as early as your mid to late thirties and last anywhere from four to twelve years! During perimenopause, you still have monthly cycles even if they are irregular. Once you've gone twelve consecutive months without a monthly cycle, you are officially in menopause.

The Body We Don't Recognize Anymore

Perimenopause symptoms are real—and they can feel like a betrayal. One day, your body seems to be working fine. The next, you're dealing with a cascade of changes that make no sense:

➤ Weight Gain: Especially around the belly, despite no changes in your diet or exercise. Hormonal shifts, particularly the drop in estrogen, affect fat storage and metabolism.

➤ Brain Fog: You forget names, misplace keys, and can't seem to finish a thought. It's frustrating and scary.

➤ Hot Flashes and Night Sweats: Sudden waves of heat that disrupt your sleep, leave you in a pool of sweat, and rob you of your confidence.

➤ Thinning hair and aging skin: Your once voluminous locks are now dry and thinning. Your hair is so thin that you can almost see your scalp in some areas. Your skin is looking thin, dry, and wrinkly.

➤ Mood Swings and Anxiety: You feel tense, sensitive, short-tempered, and prone to feeling overwhelmed. You don't feel like "you."

➤ Digestive Disturbances: Gas, bloating, constipation, heartburn, diarrhea, and sometimes a combination of all of them have disrupted your life and your happiness.

➤ Low Energy: Getting out of bed is hard. Getting through the day feels impossible.

➢ Sleep Disturbances: Even if you fall asleep, you wake up often, drenched in sweat or plagued by racing thoughts.

This list can go on and on – there are over 100 symptoms related to hormonal imbalances through the perimenopause and menopause years. These symptoms can appear over time or all at once. Over time, they make you feel like a stranger in your own skin. Emotional confusion worsens the physical pain. No one warned us that this would happen!

We were taught to expect puberty. We were warned about pregnancy. But perimenopause? That has been the silent season—until now.

The Emotional Toll: Who Am I Now?

The emotional weight of perimenopause is as real as the physical symptoms. And yet, many women feel shame for even admitting it. They suffer in silence, wondering why they can't "push through."

You might feel:

➢ Disconnected: From your body, your purpose, and your desires.

➢ Frustrated: That you can't explain how you feel. Doctors dismiss your concerns or offer only prescriptions with often horrendous side effects.

➢ Guilty: That you are irritable with your spouse or distant from your children.

➢ Invisible: As if society no longer sees you.

Perimenopause doesn't just touch your hormones—it touches your identity. Who are you, if your body doesn't feel like your own? If your emotions feel foreign? If your once-sharp mind now struggles with everyday tasks?

This is a grief few talk about. But it's real. And naming it is the first step toward healing.

Spiritual Disconnection and Awakening

For many women, perimenopause isn't just a physical or emotional shift—it's a spiritual reckoning.

You may feel disconnected from God. From your purpose. From the rhythm that once gave your life meaning. You ask questions you never asked before: *'What now?' 'Who am I, if I'm not who I used to be?' 'Is there more for me?'*

This spiritual unease can feel like a wilderness. But wilderness seasons are sacred. They are where deep transformation begins.

You are not being punished—you are being invited. Invited to slow down. To listen more deeply. To reconnect with the God who sees every sleepless night, every tear, every hot flash, every whispered prayer.

This season can deepen your faith, not destroy it. But it may require releasing old beliefs about worth and identity that no longer serve you.

You are not lost. You are being remade.

Unseen Strain: The Impact on Relationships and Marriage

A tough part of this journey is its impact on your relationships, especially with your spouse.

When communication breaks down, intimacy can feel far away. The strain often feels too much to bear. Neither of you may know what is really happening. Marriages often struggle due to unaddressed hormonal changes.

Surveys show that about 60% of divorces in couples over 40 happen during perimenopause. Love doesn't vanish. Instead, disconnection, misunderstandings, and emotional turmoil remain unspoken and unhealed.

You're not crazy for feeling distant. You're not selfish for needing space. Your partner needs to know what you're feeling. It all begins with you understanding it first.

You can rebuild connections. You can restore intimacy. But it takes knowledge, honesty, and support.

The Silent Shame of Libido Loss

Let's talk about something women often whisper—if they talk about it at all: the loss of desire.

You love your partner. You're still attracted to them. But your body doesn't respond the same. Your desire has waned, your body feels foreign, and what once brought intimacy now brings anxiety.

This is not just "in your head." Hormonal changes during perimenopause—especially the drop in estrogen and testosterone—affect lubrication, arousal, and sensation. Intimacy with your spouse can become uncomfortable, even painful. But few women feel safe saying that aloud.

You might feel broken. You might feel guilty. You might worry that your relationship will suffer.

But what if this season could bring a new level of honesty, tenderness, and connection? What if your worth wasn't measured by performance—but by presence?

Desire can return. Intimacy can evolve. But it starts by releasing the shame and choosing to speak truth—even when it's uncomfortable.

When Friendships Fade and Loneliness Sets In

There's a grief that few women anticipate in midlife—the quiet unraveling of friendships that once felt unbreakable. As we navigate perimenopause, our emotional bandwidth shifts. We no longer have the energy to people-please or maintain surface-level relationships. We crave deeper, more soul-nourishing connections.

But not everyone understands this change. Friends drift. Conversations become harder. You feel like you're outgrowing circles that once defined you—and it's lonely.

This loneliness isn't just about physical isolation. It's an emotional disconnection. It's walking into a room and wondering if anyone sees the real you anymore. It's wanting to be known and held, without judgment, in the rawness of this season.

If you've ever cried quietly after a lunch with friends who just "don't get it"… you're not alone. If you've ever pulled away because you didn't want to pretend everything's fine… I see you.

Your heart is not too much. Your need for depth is not a flaw. This season will refine your relationships—but it will also reveal the ones that were meant to stay.

When the Weight Isn't Just Physical

We often talk about weight gain in perimenopause. But the heaviest burdens women carry aren't measured by the scale.

It's the mental load of being everything to everyone. It's the emotional weight of feeling misunderstood. It's the spiritual exhaustion of carrying silent struggles for too long.

The pressure to "keep it together" is relentless. Smile for the kids. Show up for your job. Care for aging parents. And somehow, figure out how to deal with night sweats, brain fog, and unpredictable moods in between.

No wonder you're tired.

This season requires gentleness. The kind of grace that whispers: *'You're doing your best. And that's enough.'*

Let go of perfection. Let go of comparison. Let go of the inner critic who says you should have it all figured out by now.

You are not lazy. You are healing. You are not failing. You are transitioning. You are not weak. You are in a sacred transformation.

Digestive Drama and the Belly You Don't Recognize

Your belly feels bloated after every meal. Foods you once enjoyed now cause pain. Your digestion is sluggish, your jeans don't zip, and you're constantly uncomfortable.

This is one of the lesser-known symptoms of perimenopause, but it's incredibly common. Estrogen and progesterone influence gut function, and when they shift, so does your digestive rhythm.

The bloat isn't always from what you're eating. It's from how your body is handling stress, hormones, and inflammation.

Healing the gut is healing the woman. And when you nourish your digestive system, your mood, energy, and hormones begin to stabilize too.

You deserve to feel light in your body again.

When Aging Doesn't Feel Graceful

There's a harsh reality many women face in perimenopause: the feeling of aging before your time. Your joints ache, your face feels less vibrant, and your once-thick hair is now thinning in the shower drain. Your skin, once glowing, feels dull, dry, or sagging in unfamiliar places. You may stare into the mirror and wonder, *'Where did she go?'*

For a woman who's spent her life taking care of others, being admired for her beauty, or praised for her strength—it's a grieving process. You didn't expect to feel invisible. You didn't know how much your identity was wrapped up in how you felt in your own skin.

And the kicker? You're still expected to show up, to lead, to smile. Even when you haven't had a full night's sleep in months. Even when your heart is racing from a hot flash while you're trying to get dinner on the table. Even when brain fog keeps you from finishing a sentence in a meeting.

This isn't vanity. It's humanity. Your desire to feel beautiful, strong, and alive is not shallow—it's sacred.

You were never meant to suffer silently.

Perimenopause isn't just a hormonal shift—it's an emotional earthquake. And when we don't talk about it, we isolate ourselves in a struggle that is wildly common and deeply misunderstood. But when we speak it aloud—when we say, this is hard, and I'm still worthy of love and care—something powerful happens. We begin to heal.

Memory Loss and the Fear of Losing Yourself

You walk into a room and forget why. You search for words you've always known. You reread the same paragraph three times and still can't absorb it.

It's terrifying.

No one told you that memory lapses could be part of perimenopause. That brain fog could mimic early dementia. That you'd begin questioning your intelligence.

But it's not the end of your sharp mind. It's a pause—a recalibration. One influenced by stress, hormone shifts, and deep exhaustion.

You haven't lost your mind. You've just misplaced it temporarily.

Rest. Nourish. Replenish. Your clarity will return.

And in the meantime, give yourself the grace you'd offer your best friend.

The Silent Struggle with Anxiety

You've always been strong. Capable. Calm. But now, out of nowhere, your chest tightens. Your heart races. Your mind spins. You lie awake with irrational fears, obsessing over things that never used to bother you.

Welcome to the hidden link between perimenopause and anxiety.

The drop in estrogen affects serotonin—the "feel-good" hormone. Cortisol levels skyrocket, and your nervous system feels hijacked.

This anxiety doesn't always look like panic. Sometimes, it's indecision. Sometimes, it's avoiding social plans. Sometimes, it's a racing mind that won't turn off.

If this is you, breathe.

You are not crazy. You are not weak. You are responding to a storm within that deserves care, not condemnation.

There are gentle, natural ways to support your nervous system. You don't have to suffer in silence. You are worthy of peace.

Rage, Shame, and the Fear of Losing Control

One of the most unexpected symptoms of perimenopause is rage. Not just irritability—but red-hot, soul-shaking rage. The kind that boils up from nowhere over something small: someone chewing too loudly, shoes left in the hallway, a delay in traffic.

It scares you. It surprises you. And it leaves you feeling ashamed.

You wonder, yet again, *'Who am I right now?'*

This level of emotional intensity can feel like you've lost control of yourself. You apologize, cry in the bathroom, and vow to "get it together." But what if you're not broken? What if your hormones are calling for attention, not punishment?

This rage is often a cocktail of progesterone decline, cortisol overload, and years of unspoken emotional labor. It's not your fault—and it doesn't make you a bad mom, wife, or friend. It makes you human.

Let's normalize this conversation and remind each other that strong women also have breaking points. You are allowed to feel. You are allowed to get help. And you are still worthy of love in your most unglued moments.

When Sleep Becomes a Stranger

It used to be simple. You'd close your eyes and drift off. But now, sleep evades you. You lie awake for hours. You wake up drenched in sweat. Your mind races with thoughts you can't silence.

Night after night, the exhaustion compounds. You wake up tired. You move through the day in a fog. And worst of all, you feel like your body is betraying you during the time it's meant to heal.

Insomnia in perimenopause is real. It's not just poor sleep hygiene. It's not just "getting older."

Your changing hormones are disrupting your body's natural rhythms. Melatonin production dips. Cortisol rises when it shouldn't. And your nervous system forgets how to rest.

Sleep isn't a luxury. It's your lifeline. And when it's taken from you, everything suffers—your mood, your weight, your memory, your relationships.

You are not imagining this. You are not alone. And you can get restful sleep again with the right support.

Let's bring peace back to your nights. Because you deserve to wake up refreshed—and ready to live again.

Skin That Doesn't Feel Like Yours Anymore

One day, you notice it. The softness is gone. Your skin feels thinner. Drier. Crepey. Your once-youthful glow is replaced by dullness. Wrinkles deepen. Elasticity fades.

And no amount of cream seems to fix it.

What's happening isn't just external—it's hormonal. Estrogen plays a huge role in skin hydration, collagen production, and elasticity. As it declines, your skin reflects the change.

But here's what's also true: your skin tells your story.

Those fine lines? Proof of laughter. Those scars? Markers of survival. That texture? Evidence of years lived and lessons learned.

You're allowed to grieve the changes. But don't forget to celebrate the resilience in every pore. You can support your skin from the inside out—with minerals, hydration, nourishment, and rest.

You're still radiant. You always have been.

Hair Loss and the Quiet Panic It Brings

It starts with a few extra strands in the brush. Then, clumps in the shower. A receding hairline. A widening part. You run your fingers through your hair and feel the loss.

No one told you this would happen. No one warned you how deeply it would shake your confidence.

Hair loss during perimenopause is common—but that doesn't make it easy.

It feels personal. Like something sacred is being stripped away. Your identity, femininity, and youth all feel wrapped up in it.

You stare at your scalp in the mirror, hoping for change—and dreading the next wash.

But you are not alone. And you are not powerless.

Mineral imbalances, thyroid shifts, and stress all play a role. With the right tools—like HTMA testing, Biofeedback scan and support—you can nourish your scalp, rebalance your body, and reclaim growth.

Your beauty is not defined by your hair. But you are allowed to want to feel beautiful again.

Joint Pain, Stiffness, and the Fear of Growing Old Too Soon

Your knees ache. Your hips feel tight. Your fingers are stiff. Getting out of bed feels like shaking off rust.

You used to be active. Flexible. Strong.

Now, everything hurts.

Estrogen protects joints, ligaments, and cartilage. And as it declines, inflammation creeps in. Your body, once fluid, starts to feel rigid. Movement becomes a chore.

You fear you're aging faster than you should.

But there is hope. Gentle movement, anti-inflammatory foods, targeted minerals—all of these can bring relief. You don't have to accept pain as your new normal.

You are still strong. And your body is still capable of healing.

When Tears Come Without Warning

You're folding laundry, and suddenly you're crying. You hear a song from your past, and the floodgates open. You forget a grocery item, and it feels like the end of the world.

This is not weakness. This is your nervous system under pressure.

The emotional waves in perimenopause are intense. Estrogen influences mood regulation and neurotransmitters like serotonin and dopamine. When it drops, your emotional resilience drops too.

You cry more. You feel more. You may even feel numb some days.

Let those tears fall. They are cleansing. You don't have to "get it together."

You just have to be honest—and let yourself be human.

This is not the time to harden. It's the time to soften into yourself.

When Motivation Disappears

You used to be so driven. Organized. On top of things.

Now, even the simplest tasks feel monumental.

Dishes pile up. Emails go unanswered. You sit in the car staring out the window, not knowing where to begin.

This loss of motivation isn't laziness. It's not apathy. It's hormonal burnout.

When your adrenals are taxed, your minerals are depleted, and your sleep is disrupted—your brain says, I can't.

The spark will come back. But for now, lower the bar. Choose one thing. Celebrate it.

Your worth is not measured by productivity. It's measured by your presence.

And right now, being present with your healing is enough.

When You Feel Like You're Losing Your Edge at Work

You used to be sharp. Quick. Confident.

Now, you double-check everything. You hesitate before speaking. You fear you're being replaced by someone younger, more energetic.

Perimenopause in the workplace is an invisible struggle. You're expected to perform like nothing's changed, even as your body and mind scream for mercy.

This fear of irrelevance cuts deep. But you are not losing value—you are gaining wisdom.

You still belong here. And the world needs your perspective more than ever.

Speak your truth. Ask for support. Set boundaries.

You're not falling behind. You're evolving.

Grieving the Woman You Used to Be

There comes a point when you realize you're mourning someone: yourself.

Not because she's gone forever, but because her season has ended. The woman who could stay up late and wake up early. The one with thick hair and glowing skin. The one who had endless energy for everyone else.

Grief shows up quietly. In the way you hesitate before putting on a swimsuit. In the way you avoid mirrors. In the way you push through fatigue while aching for someone to say, "It's okay to rest."

It's okay to grieve. And it's okay to fall in love with the woman you are becoming.

She's softer. Wiser. Fiercer. More discerning. She knows what matters now.

This is not a loss—it's a rebirth. But first, we must honor the letting go.

The Cost of Caregiving While You're Falling Apart

Many women in midlife are part of the "sandwich generation"—caring for both children and aging parents. Add full-time jobs, financial pressure, and hormonal chaos, and it's a recipe for burnout.

You pour from a cup that's long been empty. You feel guilty for not doing enough and resentment for being expected to do it all.

And yet, you keep showing up.

But who's caring for you?

This season demands boundaries. Not as selfishness—but as survival.

Say no. Ask for help. Delegate. Rest without guilt.

The world will not fall apart when you prioritize your well-being.

You are not weak for needing rest—you are wise for honoring your limits.

The Mirror Is Not the Enemy

You've stared at your reflection and thought, I don't recognize her.

The lines, the puffiness, the tired eyes. The clothes that don't fit. The sagging where there used to be strength.

But what if you looked again—and saw the warrior?

The woman who has survived heartbreak, carried generations, and shows up again and again despite it all?

You are not less beautiful—you are more. More layered. More lived-in. More luminous.

And the mirror? It's not your enemy. It's your witness.

Look again. See her.

The Inner Critic Gets Louder—Until You Silence Her

There's a voice in your head that says:

"You're not enough."

"You're too much."

"You're aging and irrelevant."

She's harsh. She's constant. And she's lying.

Perimenopause often brings up unresolved wounds—childhood messaging, cultural expectations, old insecurities. And without realizing it, we let this inner critic become the narrator of our lives.

But you can choose a new voice. One rooted in truth:

"I am worthy of care."

"I am strong through change."

"I am becoming someone powerful."

You get to be the author now. Let grace speak louder than judgment.

A New Way to Measure Strength

In this season of change, strength is no longer about powering through or doing it all.

Strength is:

Choosing rest instead of guilt.

Saying no without explanation.

Asking for help when you need it.

Letting go of unrealistic expectations.

Nourishing your body out of love—not punishment.

Perimenopause invites us to rewrite the story of womanhood. No longer defined by hustle or perfection, but by resilience, grace, and self-respect.

You are not weak because you're tired. You're not failing because your body is shifting. You are becoming.

Your Body Is Not the Enemy

This might be the most radical truth of all: your body is not the enemy. Every symptom, every signal—it's communication. Your body is asking for your attention, your care, your compassion.

Instead of fighting her, what if you chose to partner with her?

Instead of silencing her with shame, what if you listened with curiosity?

This shift changes everything. It moves us from self-blame to self-honor. It reclaims our power.

The Power of Reconnection

One of the most beautiful gifts of perimenopause is the chance to return to yourself.

You begin to remember who you were before the world told you who to be. You start honoring your body instead of fighting it. You begin to hear your intuition more clearly. You rediscover dreams you thought were buried.

This reconnection is not a luxury—it's a necessity.

Start small. Read a devotional for women. Journal for five minutes in the morning. Walk in silence. Stroll in nature. Breathe deeply and stretch. Say kind things to yourself in the mirror.

These tiny acts of reconnection create a ripple effect. They awaken the spark. They remind you that you matter, too.

And as you come back home to yourself, you show other women that they can, too.

Why Women Don't Seek Help—and Why That Has to Change

So many women don't seek help until they're at their breaking point. Why?

Because they have been dismissed before.

Because they think it's "just aging."

Because they're used to putting everyone else first.

But the truth is: you can't pour from an empty cup. And your symptoms are not a life sentence—they're a signal.

It's time to stop ignoring, stop guessing and start listening!

Hope Is Possible

The best news? Balance is possible. Peace is possible. Even joy—yes, joy—is possible again.

When your hormones begin to stabilize through nourishment, rest, and support, your thoughts shift. You begin to see clearly again. You laugh more. You breathe deeper. You feel like the woman you always hoped you'd be— not the one you left behind.

This isn't the end of your story. It's the moment everything turns.

You are not just surviving this season. You are being transformed by it.

And on the other side? A woman fully alive.

Let This Be the Season You Choose You

Perimenopause will change you. But it doesn't have to break you.

- ➤ Let this be the season you:

- ➤ Say yes to rest

- ➤ Say no without guilt

- ➤ Nourish your body without punishment

- ➤ Trust your intuition

- ➤ Let go of what no longer serves you

- ➤ This is not the end. It's your reawakening.

You are still her. You are still worthy. You are still radiant.

And the next chapter of your life can be the most powerful one yet.

Let's Talk About Confidence: Rebuilding It from the Inside Out

Confidence doesn't come from the scale, the mirror, or external validation. It comes from alignment.

And perimenopause, while painful, is the ultimate invitation to realign with who you are. With what you value. With how you want to show up.

Confidence is built in the quiet moments:

When you choose rest without guilt.

When you speak truth instead of pretending.

When you look in the mirror and say, "I'm still here."

You don't need to become a new woman. You just need to come back home to the one you've always been.

The Way Forward: Healing, Balance, and Hope

This is the part of the journey where the light begins to return.

You can heal from perimenopause, and it doesn't need a one-size-fits-all method. Listen to your body. Understand your symptoms. Then, create a personalized path forward.

I use a holistic, root-cause approach. This method doesn't just hide your symptoms. It shows the reasons behind them. We use tools like Biofeedback Scan Technology and HTMA, or Hair Tissue Mineral Analysis and follow our transformational process called the Health & Harmony System. Biofeedback scans reveal the root causes of stress in your organs, glands, and systems. They provide a clear picture of your stressors. This helps us understand how to support your body and find relief. The HTMA (Hair Tissue Mineral Analysis) test reveals essential insights into your mineral levels, metabolism, and stress patterns. When we see these patterns, we can start restoring what's out of balance.

But this journey isn't just about tests. It's about nurturing every part of you. We collaborate to make easy, sustainable changes in nutrition, movement, rest, and mindset. These areas all affect your hormones and healing.

Here's what healing can look like:

➢ Waking up with energy instead of dread.

➢ Feeling confident in your clothes again.

➢ Maintaining a clear mindset and managing stress with greater composure.

➢ Reconnecting with your spouse or partner creates open communication and renewed intimacy.

➢ Feeling like YOU again.

And it's not just possible. It's happening for women every single day. Women received the message that they were "fine," despite their evident struggles. Women felt dismissed and discouraged. They chose to find the answers that were essential to them.

You can reclaim your clarity, your peace, your vibrance. And it starts with believing you deserve it!

You Are Not Alone...There is Hope

Sister, I see you.

I see the woman who's exhausted and confused. The woman wondering where her sparkle went. The woman afraid that life will never feel good again.

Let me remind you: there is so much hope!

What you're experiencing is part of a profound transition, but it's not the end of your story. In fact, it can be the most powerful turning point of your life. This isn't about "going back to who you were." It's about becoming the most aligned and empowered version of who you are today.

You are not too far gone. You are not broken. You are not alone!

There is a path. There is a plan. And there are people—myself included—ready to walk with you.

Let this be your invitation to rise. To reclaim your health, your joy, and your story.

Because the best version of you isn't lost. She's waiting. And she's worth fighting for!

About the Author

April Ranard is a Christian Life & Certified Holistic Health Coach. She helps Christian women over 35 understand & navigate the confusing symptoms of perimenopause, menopause and hormonal imbalances. With more than a decade of experience, April offers a comprehensive virtual approach that includes personalized coaching, VIP days, group support, specific hormone testing, and lifestyle changes no matter where you are in the world. She provides women with clarity & lasting transformation in a supportive and compassionate environment.

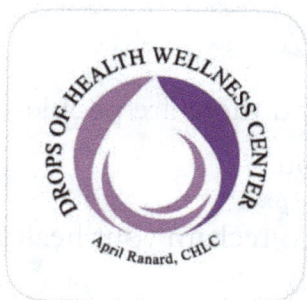

April helps women regain energy, balance hormones, lose weight, and so much more. Her signature program and wellness tools help women reconnect with vibrant lives. She founded Drops of Health Wellness and founded and hosts The Midlife Reset ~ Hormones, Weight & Energy - Simplified podcast.

Visit April at www.dropsofhealthwellnesscenter.com to book a free Midlife Strategy Call and get your free Hormone Health Habit Tracker to start your journey back to yourself.

AN APPLE A DAY IS A START... BUT WHAT ELSE IS ON YOUR PLATE?

JOYCE B. NYAIRO (DR. FEEL GOOD)

Certified Health & Lifestyle Coach | Founder of Amazing
Balance International Group, Creator of *Joyce's Choices*
Healing Kitchen

CHAPTER FIVE

AN APPLE A DAY IS A START... BUT WHAT ELSE IS ON YOUR PLATE?

Joyce B. Nyairo (Dr. Feel Good)

Certified Health & Lifestyle Coach | Founder of Amazing Balance International Group, Creator of Joyce's Choices Healing Kitchen

Introduction

The age-old saying, "An apple a day keeps the doctor away," carries timeless wisdom — but in today's fast-paced, overburdened world, it takes more than one apple to sustain health and wholeness.

True health is about life balance: nourishing not just our bodies, but also our hearts, minds, and spirits. In

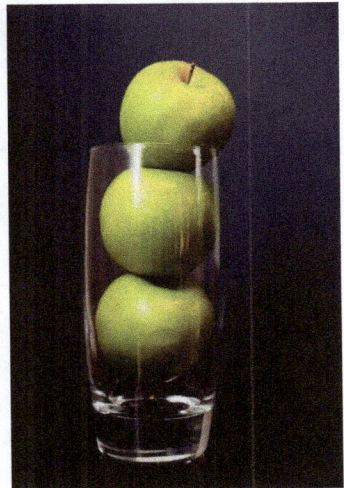

this chapter, I invite you to reflect on what else is on your plate — both literally and figuratively — and to consider how your daily choices shape your long-term health, peace, and joy.

The Power of Daily Choices

Health is built one decision at a time. The Bible reminds us in **3 John 1:2 (KJV):**

"Beloved, I wish above all things that thou mayest prosper and be in health, even as thy soul prospereth."

This scripture highlights the inseparable connection between physical health and spiritual well-being. What we consume in spirit, body, and mind ultimately determines the quality of our lives.

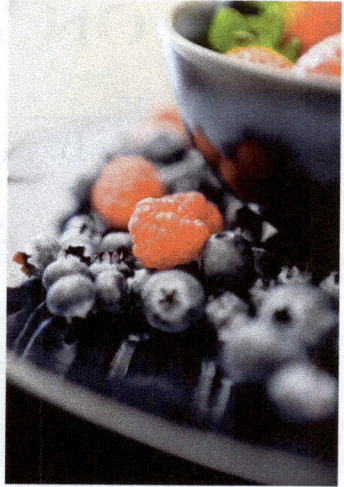

Health is built one choice at a time. The Bible offers timeless wisdom:

- **Proverbs 17:22 (KJV)** – "A merry heart doeth good like a medicine." → *A joyful heart brings healing and good health.*

- **John 10:10 (KJV)** – "I am come that they might have life, and that they might have it more abundantly." → *Jesus came to give us abundant life in every aspect.*

- **Genesis 1:29 (KJV)** – "I have given you every herb bearing seed… to you it shall be for meat." → *God's original plan was plant-based nourishment.*

- **1 Corinthians 6:19-20 (KJV)** – "Your body is the temple of the Holy Ghost… therefore glorify God in your body." → *Our bodies are sacred and deserve care and respect.*

What Else Is on Your Plate?

Beyond food, our plates hold stress, relationships, purpose, faith, work, and emotional well-being. Many illnesses don't begin in the kitchen — they start in the heart and mind. A balanced, fulfilling life requires tending to both our physical needs and our inner world.

Life Nourishment: Primary and Secondary Foods

During my training at the *Institute for Integrative Nutrition (IIN)*, I discovered a life-changing concept:

Primary Food: Relationships, career, physical activity, spirituality, joy, creativity, and self-care.

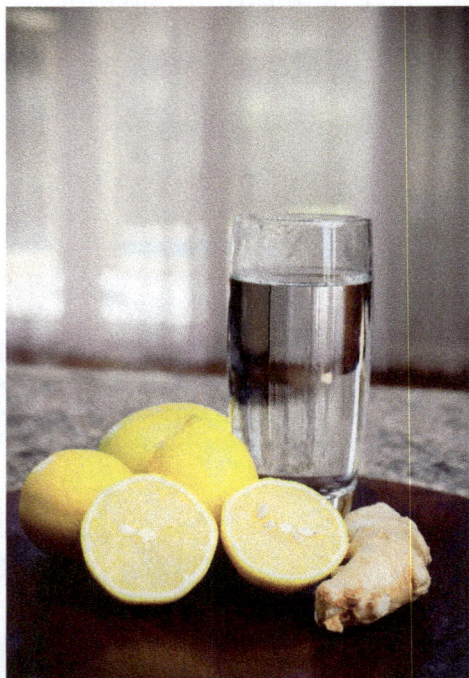

Secondary Food: The actual food on your plate.

When Primary Food is nourishing and satisfying, your craving for unhealthy Secondary Food decreases. I am forever grateful to IIN for this transformative framework.

My Journey to Amazing Balance

After 17 intense years working at the *International Monetary Fund* (IMF), stress and overwork took a toll on my health. Chronic fatigue, stress-related illnesses, and emotional burnout forced me to reevaluate my life.

I left my career prematurely, embarking on a healing journey through nutrition, stress management, faith, and natural living. That transformational path inspired me to create Amazing Balance International Group — a holistic lifestyle company that helps others reclaim their vitality and purpose.

The AMAZE Formula

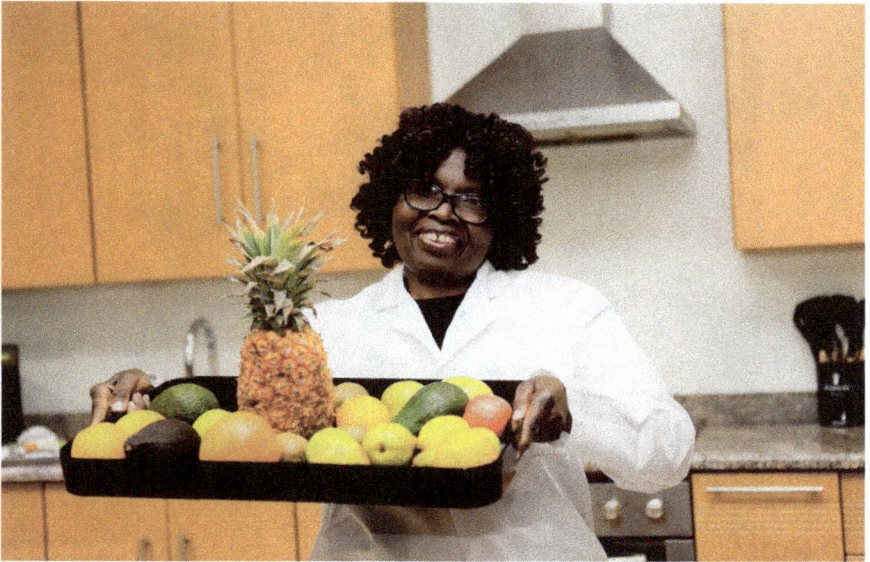

At the heart of my philosophy is *AMAZE*, a *five-pillar formula* for life balance and personal wellness:

- • Accountability
- • Management of thoughts and habits
- • Attraction through positive mirroring behaviors
- • Zest for life
- • Energy alignment through nutrition, movement, and spiritual connection

This formula serves as the foundation for every coaching program, speaking engagement, and client relationship that I nurture through **Amazing Balance International Group**.

The Divine Health Prescription

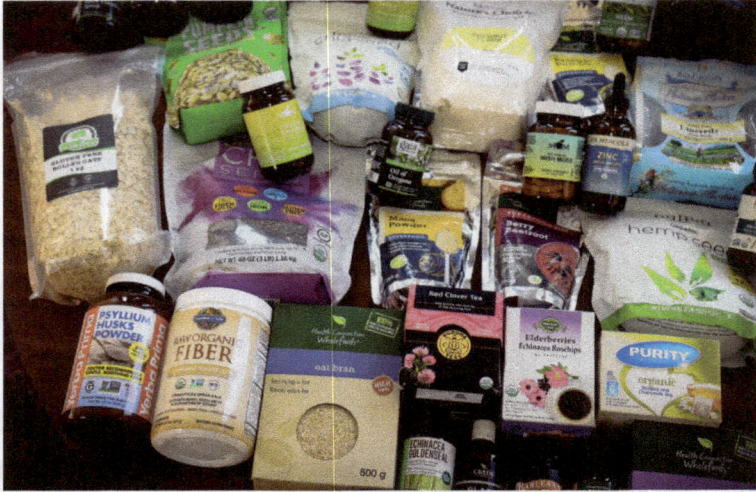

The Bible declares in Proverbs 17:22:

> *"A merry heart doeth good like a medicine."*

Health is sacred.

My Divine Health Prescription includes:

✔ Purpose-driven living

✔ Plant-based, whole foods

✔ Daily physical movement

✔ Quality rest

✔ Healthy, nurturing relationships

✔ Spiritual connection and worship

Foods to Embrace

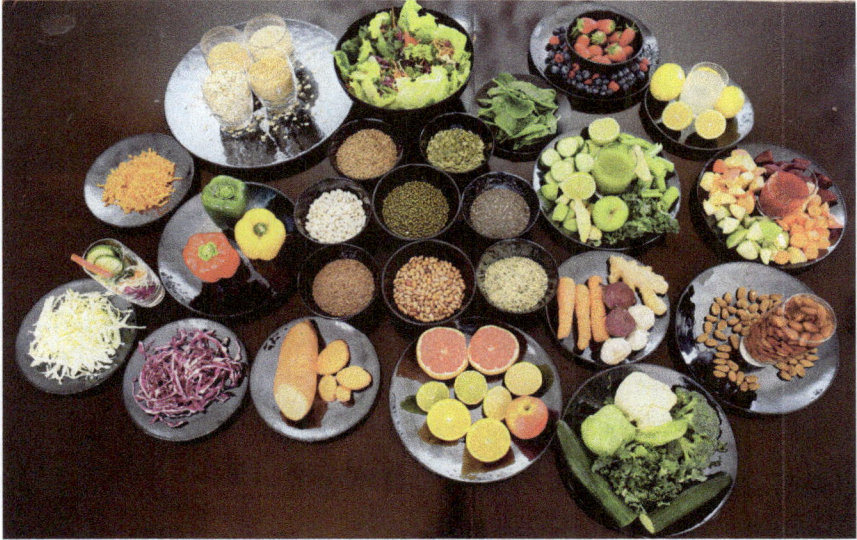

- Fresh fruits and vegetables (apples, berries, greens)
- Herbs and spices (ginger, garlic, turmeric)
- Whole grains (wild rice, quinoa, millet)
- Legumes (lentils, black beans, chickpeas)
- Herbal teas
- Clean, pure water

Foods to Limit

- • Processed and packaged foods
- • Refined sugars and artificial sweeteners
- • Excess salt, fried foods, and processed meats
- • Artificial additives
- • Overconsumption of animal products

Life Balance Check-In

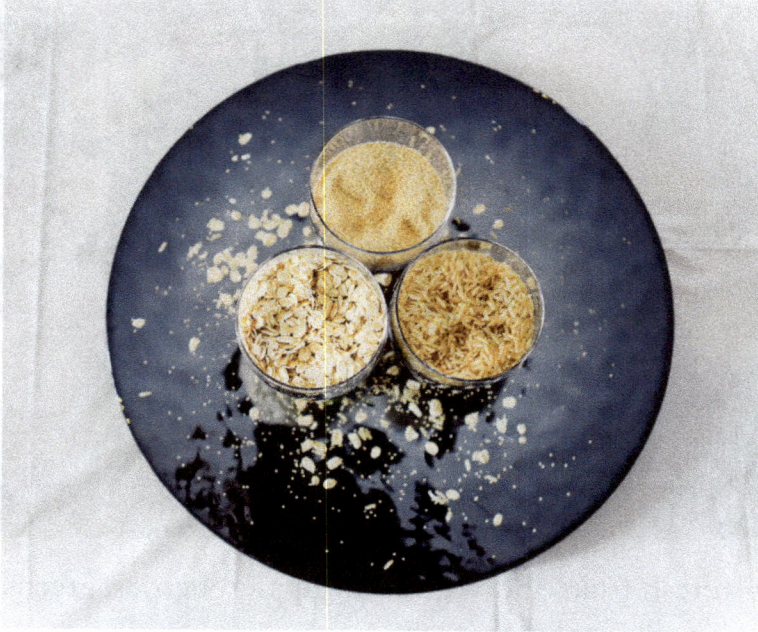

I encourage you to regularly pause and reflect:

- Are my relationships healthy and life-giving?
- Are my relationships healthy?
- Am I living on purpose?
- Do I practice gratitude and joy?
- How's my sleep, movement, and spiritual life?
- Do I feel energized and aligned?

Health is more than food — it's about wholeness.

Conclusion

An apple a day is a good start. But abundant health comes from what else is on your plate — emotionally, spiritually, physically, and relationally.

As John 10:10 (KJV) reminds us:

> *"I am come that they might have life, and*
> *that they might have it more abundantly."*

Let's choose abundance in every area of life — one intentional choice at a time.

Closing Blessing

May you prosper in health, peace, and purpose as
you nourish your body, mind, and spirit.

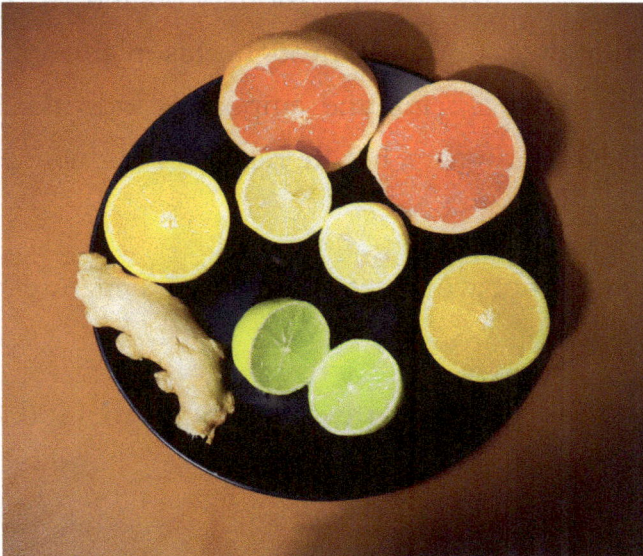

About the Author

Founder and President, Amazing Balance International Group, LLC

"Balancing Life, Love, and Language"

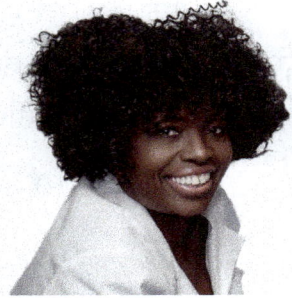

Born in the vibrant village of Kisii, Kenya, Joyce B. Nyairo is a multilingual global explorer whose life journey weaves together a rich tapestry of culture, wellness, and holistic living. Her diverse experiences across continents bring a soul-nourishing essence to the world of nutrition and personal development.

A Certified Health & Lifestyle Coach, Organic Nourishment Chef, Protocol and Etiquette Consultant, and international speaker, Joyce is the visionary behind Amazing Balance International Group. Through this platform, she champions holistic well-being and empowers individuals to achieve balance in spirituality, health, relationships, work, and finances.

At the core of her work lies AMAZE, a signature five-pillar philosophy built around:

1. **Accountability** – We are accountable to God, our parents, and ourselves.

2. **Management** – We must steward our bodies, money, spiritual lives, and more responsibly.

3. **Attraction** – Wise management attracts others and helps build your tribe.

4. **Zest** – With clarity comes joy and motivation for life.

5. **Energy** – Real health flows from spiritual, physical, relational, work, and financial vitality.

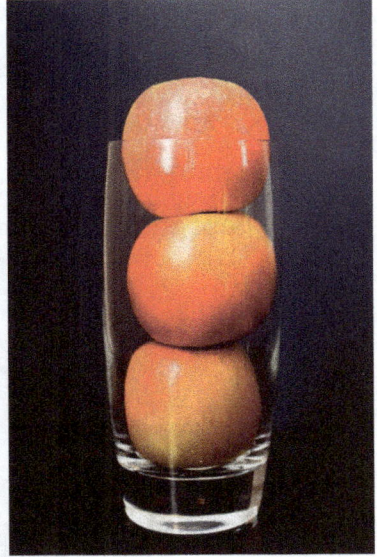

Joyce's Signature Programs:

- Joyce's Choices Healing Kitchen
- 28-Day Clean Slate Detox Program
- Weight Wellness Blueprint
- High Five Heart Health Program
- Pre-Diabetes and Diabetes Management Program

Her professional background includes impactful work at the International Monetary Fund (IMF) and the International Agency for Research on Cancer (IARC) in Lyon, France, where she gained invaluable leadership and advocacy experience.

Fluent in Kisii, Kiswahili, English, and French—and currently learning Spanish—Joyce has traveled to over 40 countries and once flew aboard the Concorde. Her mission: to help others find harmony in life, love, and language, and to coach them into becoming fluent in the language of holistic well-being.

Contact Joyce B. Nyairo

Email: joyce@theamazingbalance.com

Website: www.theamazingbalance.com

Twitter: @AmazingBalance

Facebook: Amazing Balance LLC

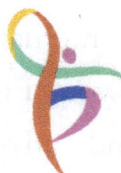

Amazing Balance
INTERNATIONAL GROUP

HAVE U MET U?

Your Masterpiece Life Awaits

ELIZABETH VILLALPANDO ELLISON

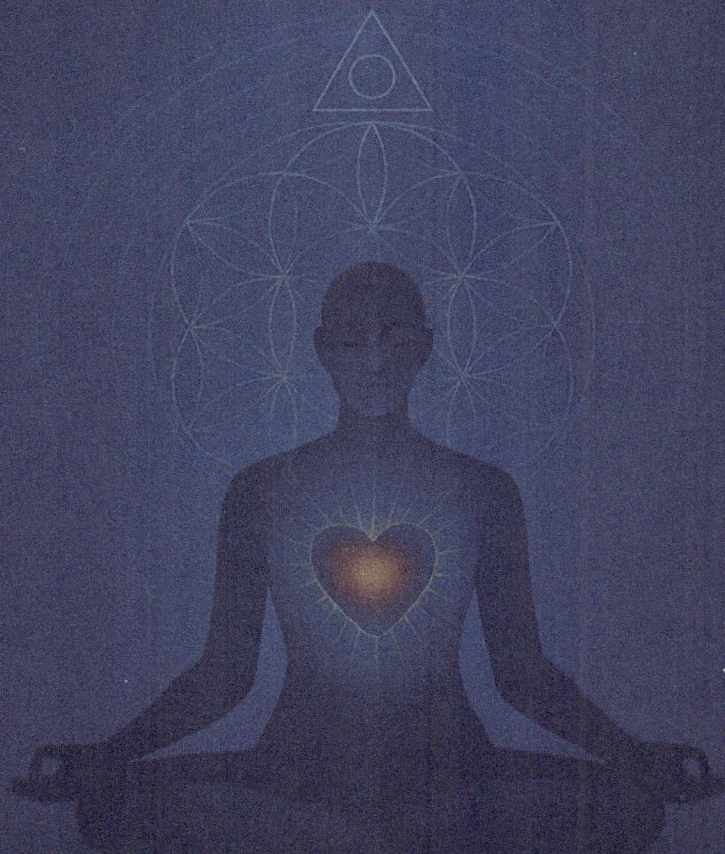

In loving memory of my parents and baby sisters.
Thank you for the countless joys, abundant love, and shared
laughter that continue to illuminate my path and inspire me
to help others find their own light.

CHAPTER SIX

HAVE U MET U?
YOUR MASTERPIECE LIFE AWAITS

Elizabeth Villalpando Ellison

Finding Your Way Home to Yourself

To master yourself you will first need to identify the foolish side of you. **Be** able to be **U**. The subject matter here at hand is no joke. It's serious ~ our choices are. Life these days is so different than when I was 5, yet at the same time it isn't. No matter what era, it's still the same, and will still be the same when it comes to the effects that when a person feels disconnected from the rest of the other humans and their social environment, the results can be devastating.

So, I will travel with you, briefly, as this is a short chapter, from the struggles and angsts of life, the source of our daily living, that can turn to addictions, and then to healing, discovering truth, and achieving prosperity. I will trace a path from the despair and self-destruction of the source of how I discovered where my addictions came from. And what has led me to become a vibrant, holistic recovery-rooted person in self-awareness and authenticity. I first want to publicly apologize to those who traveled that road with me. I make every moment of every day now to leave a healthy legacy.

The Insidious Nature of Our Slow Destructions

Let's start by framing addiction as one of the slowest forms of suicide, and you will capture highlights of its insidious nature. Habits, feelings, perceptions, once built within my core, hidden as what I thought were strengths, but were actually permissions to slowly give away my integrity and to deny myself self-care. You will hopefully see a parallel for yourself - and pull back from what we refer to as "*stinking thinking*" in the rooms of recovery ~ to becoming aware of which of your thoughts have permitted you to stand true on your convictions, to not participate in behaviors that cause your soul sadness. To instead put thoughtful emphasis on discovering the "truth of self." Then develop and design a redemptive, empowering process with the inclusion of confidence, competence, contentment, and joy as your outcomes reflect a multidimensional healing connection with yourself that goes beyond mere balance of thought and into a thriving life. Prosperity in body, mind, heart, and soul underscores your comprehensive transformation, appealing to you seeking both practical and spiritual growth.

Human BEings in a World of Human DO

You are human **BE**ings in a world of human **DO**. You will find I like emphasizing the roots of words within words for added attention, with the goal of intentionally helping guide you.

I use the letter, **U**, to emphasize that when the "you" of us is full like a goblet/cup/vessel, and when shaped like a "**U**" we can receive and then can hold things that can be poured into ourselves, and out of it to fill up those around us. My life has proven that I am here to help **U** learn how to fill U up, then when beneficial pour yourself into the lives of others with positivity so that their "cups runneth over" also. That is an Old English phrase that you can Google, if you choose. With that I would love to invite you to take a moment and choose and think about one of the first rules I have learned. How we learn to be able to hear our Selves, and know your Self. Learn to be still and listen, beginning each day, and ending each day.

What are you going to "make" of your day today? Are you in autopilot, or intentionally designing them? How is it going to affect others, or are you going to take some time and just BE, by yourself and turn everything off and allow your 'SELF' to be?

Silent. Quiet. Still.

The Power of Stillness

To **BE** comfortable in that silence, all those moments of silence, and **BE** that person that is guided into the stillness of darkness, into finding the deep places, into your soul and not afraid of the dark. Unless you embrace the moments of quiet reflection, you cannot and will NOT be happy and content in your many moments in the light. EVER.

You WILL BE that person who cannot BE THE PERSON THAT CAN BE IN A ROOM FULL OF OTHER PEOPLE AND "JUST BE THE PERSON", that is U. Singularly "U."

Contented Wholeness.

For me, our Creator placed within us all how to **BE** creators. All these things matter. You being allowed to develop a **U** that is connected, healthy, and prosperous in your environment is a must. Most important to your "**U**" is that you understand the power of choice. Without it, whether you choose to be a hermit living alone in the mountains or a Wall Street investor surrounded by other people constantly, if **U** do not know what makes you, **U**, you will disconnect. Not feel significant in life and the living of it. The result is catastrophic. **U** are designed to choose what contentment means and create it. Hold that and you can be resilient and find joy, in any situation, in any set of circumstances, and still have enough joy to offer to others.

We are human **BE**ings in a world of **DO**. The truth of that matter is that I must, and you're "I" must, be able to learn to sit still with yourself and be able to determine who you are before you go and be with others so that **U** do not cause harm or discord, chaos, the majority of the time. Do we ever completely heal… as long as we are alive, we will need connection with others to "get through to the other side of things". There is great joy in that. But here is something to help you maintain highs longer… even hermits interact with the other animals.

The Battery Analogy

Think about this:

You ever hear of someone in their mid 30's or 40's, seemingly healthy in all respects; and they went to bed one night and didn't wake up. Heart attack. No seeming explanation is known because they are no longer available to ask the questions that would explain the actual reason. When you use something that has a battery, the battery gets used up. **U** are an energy source.

If you charge the device that is using the battery without turning the device off, both the battery and the device wear out faster.

When the device and the battery, and all its systems are never allowed to rest, they break down.

This is true for your body, mind, emotions, soul, and spirit. This shows up in your whirlwinds of **BE** and **DO**. This chaos often manifests as resentment for doing even the little daily tasks of your life as a mother, father, brother, sister, coworker. It wears and depresses, and you seek out quick fixes to feel, "better" ... I "need" a (cigarette, drink, pill, sex, ...). The choice of "*want*" vs "*need*" becomes distorted.

How a person sees themselves in the world determines how they take care of, or don't take care of, themselves. This carries over to how they can or may not be able to care well for others, also.

The Eye of the Hurricane

For the discussion here, I want you to picture each human being in the eye of a hurricane. The eye of a hurricane is one of the most still places a person can find themselves on this planet. So, you're in the eye of the hurricane all around you will see everything that the hurricane's winds have picked up in its path. Picture everything in your life swirling around you, and close your eyes and think:

How do I manage everything in my life?

Are you trying to be everything that *life* wants **U** to BE? With or without children next to you and everything that is **U** which are your responsibilities? Have you created a protective bubble that you hope is going to be enough to protect you but instead all this swirling has picked up cars, and jobs, and furniture, and money, and animals, and other people are swirling as school or work time starts ticking because time is a part of all of this and there are deadlines to meet, and bills to pay… are you in contentment or chaos? I hope you have found your contentment in all these. **U** can have that joy in gratitude.

The Power of Feelings

How we feel is the most important determining element in all relevance to every decision we make. Period. Therefore, how you choose to "be with your feelings" will determine how you move within, and without, your life, and every life, that is a part of your life.

Example0: If you do not know yourself, you cannot know the type of people you will best match up with either. My **Have U Met U** (HUMU) relationships coaching and consulting has a very simple tool to help you 'see' your way to what you truly feel to get clarity on this, and so much more.

Let's break this down. That means that if you do not understand why you feel the feeling that you choose to feel in any given moment, **U** will not be the master of your life.

If you do not Master yourself, you will become a Slave to yourself."—Elizabeth Villalpando Ellison

The Choice is Yours

The best and most hopeful part of all of this is that **U** get to choose each and every second what mastery means for you. You are your own "Self", which is an island owned by **U**. There are outside influences, but you "get to choose" how your life will affect you. Truly, yes.

How do I know this is possible? I know because I have endured many, many, many things. From being molested while still in diapers, to numerous near-death experiences, to physically being kicked off the bed during a miscarriage because I was disturbing the baby father's sleep, to name a half a drop of a flood of such instances. I did not realize that each one of those situations took a piece of me and became a shadow voice telling me I didn't matter as much as others-if there was a school that teaches this I would have known better. My coaching is that school. I needed to learn:

"Just because things are the way they are, does not mean that is how they should be."

Albert Einstein was known to say,

"The world, as we have created it, is a process of our thinking. It cannot be changed without changing our thinking."

Knowing my why and my what and how, **BE**ing me, has kept me alive. Our souls are amazing.

But I want more than to just live. I have been with many people as their souls left their bodies. They have an effervescent light to them. One was my fiancé who spoke to me without words. Some as their souls returned by helping them see their Self in those final moments. I love showing you how to shine your brightest.

Chaos need not be a mental diagnosis, but resilience training for managing *e-motion*. Your *e-motions* are the energy from what our values and beliefs trigger in our body and brain's processing of them, and are triggered sometimes physically first, but can be trained with intention of thought. You can choose to heal many things by intentional choice.

I have also mastered holding back my emotions in life-or-death moments where adding even one ounce of emotion would have meant the difference between life and death. I have the scar on my face from the pistol that proves this isn't theoretical.

People ask me how I smile despite what I've been through. When my stepfather came home in blackout drunkenness, feeling justified in his self-hatred, I learned if I maintained calm with no expression, it distracted the alcohol spirit demon in him to pause and lose energy, taking attention away from his prey. Us. Perhaps life isn't so dramatic when we master our choices.

People say I shouldn't have gone through that, and they're right. But here's the truth about hard times: while we work to change things from what they are to what they should be, I've been able to alter many outcomes from negative to positive with that ability.

Gratitude I'm alive to make mistakes and repair them another day. But during perimenopause and menopause, I lost that edge in my personal life—falling back into codependence while still coaching others out of theirs. It's been a tough 30 years, but worth it. I now have a much more compassionate perspective and can help others with greater understanding. Plus, I've spent 20 years being coached by experts. Though my biggest personal breakthroughs have been recent—it wasn't until I made one of my biggest mistakes that I made the largest shift in my **BE**ing, truly releasing my codependency and victim mindset.

Be Honest with Yourself

If you've lived hard, get a life coach who has been through more than you but is living well, by your standards. It is harder to claim victimhood then, and you'll transform faster.

Let them show you how you feel about having Mastery of your life. Whether or not you understand your beliefs, and you will determine whether or not you *"get to"* be *"U"*. How you speak to you and string those words together can be heard better by others because we get good at lying to ourselves. Habits become comforts. To be the intentional master of words you use when you speak to yourself is critical to the outcome and how you will feel during and after an event, and how others feel about you during and after. Have you said things **U** wish you hadn't? I recently made a huge mistake in that area with a family member, and I teach the value of saying nothing more than what needs to be said. Great process. But I bit myself in my own behind.

"Being able to be honest with yourself is the basis for how you 'can be' honest with others."

Example: Can you show up in a bathing suit without covering parts? With or without six-pack abs, be confident with how you are? How do you get there if this isn't natural, and why isn't it? *"Learn to become your own best friend"* and you'll find contentment in the **BE** of **U**. Anywhere, any time.

Do you need to find someone to be perfectly honest with? Fortunately, it's getting easier to be human, having human feelings and making mistakes. But too many feel there is no purpose. As long as you're alive, your purpose is to be you for all of us. **Suicide is permanent.* I came close during my miscarriage while allowing myself to be abused and feeling embarrassed. I'm so grateful I stayed, found true love, though deceased. I "get to" live better than imagined because of resilience.

Designing Your Success

Have you ever known people that seemingly have nothing but are completely content?

The best part of that statement is that you can too:

I love guiding clients into the, Design "*who*" you are and what "highly successful" means to your **U**, *by your own choice*. That is what makes life so absolutely fabulous! That you are supposed to design U. Not anyone else. Just U, you. That is the ultimate key. **BE**ing your own Best Friend.

When you decide to stand looking at all that you are and how you are going to be and take the time to evaluate and commit to being the person you design as yourself, no matter what else happens, then you can **BE**, *content with + in, and with + out + anywhere = Gratitude + Joy = Happiness*

You will not "feel" discomfort, you will be comfortable "in your skin" as the saying is often used.

No Chaos. No longer seeking drama to fill up an empty space in you and to stop you from being bored. No *dis-ease*. Released from addictive behaviors. Like over-eating or eating instant gratitude foods. And yes, you can eat healthy no matter your finances.

Too many people get into grief, or 12 Step, or other recovery programs trade one addiction for the addition of unhealthy eating. Diabetes, high-blood pressure, thyroid issues, etcetera. In programs for living with habits for death. Slow form of suicide. These are choices.

Simple Truths

Life is actually very simple. There are simple truths in life. The ability to be resilient comes from lived experiences, not perfect conditions. Remember, I offer you to make a difference in your own life:

> *"A difference, to be a difference, you must make a difference" is a philosophical American and Asian yin and yang concept."*

My life's purpose: To make a positive difference. I learned what not to do first, more than I would have liked to. But I understand the struggle better than if I hadn't done things wrong first. Got me off my high horse of thinking I had all the answers when I hadn't finished overcoming myself yet.

This book about *Collective Wisdom of Body and Soul* offers you several ways to achieve yours and is ultimately about solutions. Where your challenges are, there are also joys in finding your answers and opportunities to guide yourselves and others to your best selves.

The FQ3C System

As mentioned, I've developed a successful coaching process called **Have U Met U** (HUMU), featuring an assessment tool called FQ3C. This revolutionary behavioral tracking model transforms clients' awareness of their internal and external systems much faster than I had prayed to find, achieving in 90 days what used to take 9 months or more, even with ADHD, PTSD, and Autistic clients.

The results speak for themselves: clients are asking to pay me more monthly, and my most challenging case recently sent me $300, saying:

"It's Coach Appreciation Day ~ I want to show you how much I see my growth, especially now that you've added FQ3C!"

How does FQ3C work?

The biggest challenge with using assessments, quizzes, or tests with clients is wondering: Are they telling the truth? Right?

This tool eliminates that concern! It encourages clients to answer truthfully ~ with pride ~ because they're excited to see how they really scored. And they don't want to go back and change answers; they want to improve on the next round as is designed.

It puts the proverbial mirror of our behaviors right in front of us and guides you to see what is holding you back, both internally, and externally. It provides clear communication with yourself to achieve your goals and also improves communication with others. It improves your logic.

FQ3C is the GPS that you use to get to anything you ever want in life. Imagine a driver with a child in the back seat. The child is always wanting to know where they are and how long it will take to get there. You can solve this by teaching the child to read the GPS and just watch them quickly desire to be able to drive. This is what all professionals want - clients who drive their own development, so we can be there as a resource to polish their incredible growth.

Using **FQ3C** and coaching myself, I'm improving exponentially in everything. It feels like my brain's left and right sides are integrating and supporting each other. The voices in my head now speak reason, helping my "*Shadow Voices*" to come into the light so we can work things out - they simply transform into positive allies.

The Orchard of Experience: Roots of Resilience

Resilience isn't something you reach for on a shelf or locate solely in clinical definitions.

It's the way you live through recovery and change.
It's how you respond to misfortune—not once, but over and over.

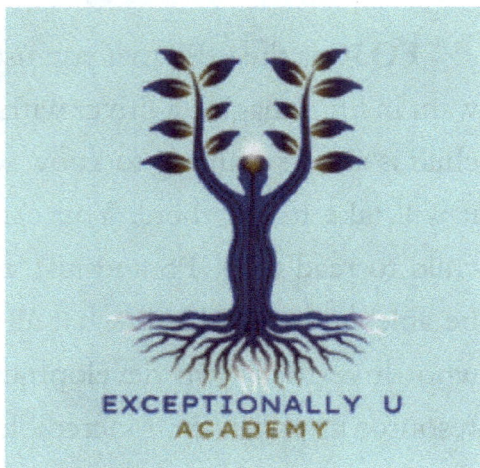

EXCEPTIONALLY U
ACADEMY

Living it—truly wearing resilience in the mud and sun of an imperfect life—is both art and science.

My own orchard was seeded in loving struggle, tremendous curiosity, and, yes, a kaleidoscope of chaos.

I was the girl who daydreamed with philosophers inside my head, wishing I could sit at the knee of Socrates or hear the whispered wisdom of elders long gone.

Instead, I competed head-to-head with older brothers and was shaped by a mother who taught me that "your better best" should be your baseline—that people shouldn't see you sweat.

But *perfectionism* isn't healthy when it convinces you that you're not good enough.

It *feeds fear of failure.*

And that fear grows when punishment replaces guidance—when discipline comes through yelling or physical correction, instead of direction and love.

Our kitchen table was a contradiction.

We talked about healthy food, healthy competition, morals, and values.

But also: *"Mix me a Bourbon & Water—or Scotch on the Rocks."*

Being able to make "the perfect drink" for my mom and her parents was oddly a badge of honor—two clashing messages about what creates wellbeing.

Their first round with alcoholism was strangely… inspirational.

They noticed irritability creeping in—a change from their usual connection.

They weren't sleeping well. One drink had become two or three. They couldn't go to bed without finishing their glass. They started drinking as soon as they got home.

And then—they stopped. Just like that.

It worked, until it didn't again.

What I've learned is this:

Addiction is selfishness.

And selfishness is not love—it's the ego's conditional love.

Conditional love plants seeds of insecurity, the kind that finds a remote, dark corner in the body, waiting…

Waiting for that one moment that zaps a buried memory awake—like a Whack-a-Mole—demanding all your attention.

The Tricycle Escape

From a tricycle adventure at age three and ending up at the local police station I learned that breaking a main rule wasn't diminished by altruistic ideals. It originally started as me wanting to show my mom that I could ride my brother's tricycle. I waited until she fell asleep to sneak out and practice riding it. It was the first time I broke one of her rules. Don't leave the house without me with you. Period. My original plan was to just ride from the steps to the sidewalk back and forth. I ended up blocks away. I learned that I had resilience in being able to identify how to be safe, but I also began my journey on compromising my integrity—a path to addiction.

This was the beginning of letting down my common sense of values and beliefs and of being sure to only do what was in my best interests, in spite of desires for instant gratification.

Unfortunately, that was not pointed out well enough.

What I offer you is to consider that you are the difference in your world. You, as an entity within yourself, make choices every moment you are alive.

Every stumble, every near miss, shapes your belief in *"the difference that makes a difference."* If anything resonates, I hope it's this: every quirk, every questionable decision, every internal debate—they make you. Don't let them break you.

HUMU FQ3C them.

Breaking the Cycle: 32 Years of Recovery

How did I finally get here? I just took my 67th turn around the sun, and 32 years consecutively without turning to mood and mind-altering substances. WOW. Finally. I started the recovery journey in 1980. It is now 2025. The math speaks for itself. I hadn't learned all my choices lead to the

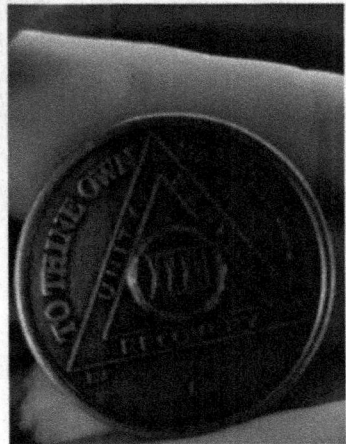

differences I wanted in my world. I am no longer a victim. I can leave or stay, but if I want change, it is my choice to be the change.

Learning from Family Patterns

I have lived 41 years since my Grandpa, who made it to age eighty in 1984, passed away from overeating. Here's the dichotomy: my parental household was based on Adele Davis's "*Let's Cook It Right*" cookbook series. We knew about healthy eating, yet addiction still found its way in.

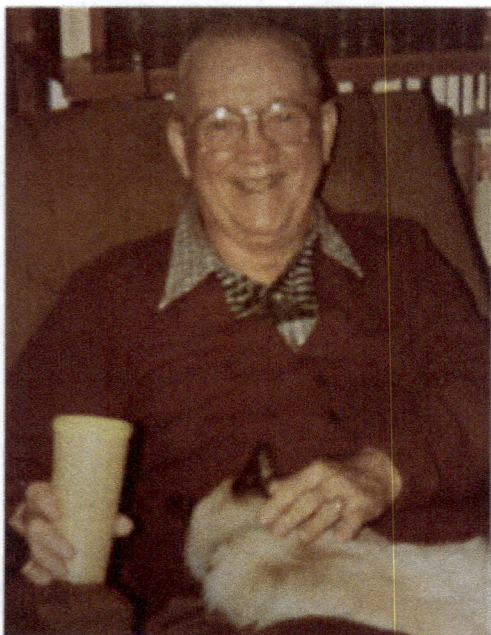

When my grandfather was hospitalized for a stroke from a poor diet, I visited him, and he recommitted to healthy eating. I called regularly and was told they were eating plain yogurt with granola, local honey and bee pollen, sourdough toast, fresh fruit, and only one egg. He was trimming down; his golf game was improving! Then I got busy, calls became less frequent, and he relapsed.

What I've learned is this:

If someone in your life is struggling, regular check-ins can be life changing. I offer this in my work—and every good recovery process includes aftercare and open-door support. Drop-ins are always welcome.

How does that apply to you?

We all have the power to be someone's support system. When I was at my lowest, one call could've changed my choices.

That's why I make it a point to reach out—even to the quieter, overlooked people in the room. I've seen those simple calls grow confidence and connection. Every time. I've been thanked. "You don't understand, no one calls me. I give out my number…

It only takes 5–10 minutes. And it matters. Every time.

Tip #1: Master Yourself or Become a Slave

"If you don't Master yourself you will become a slave to yourself."

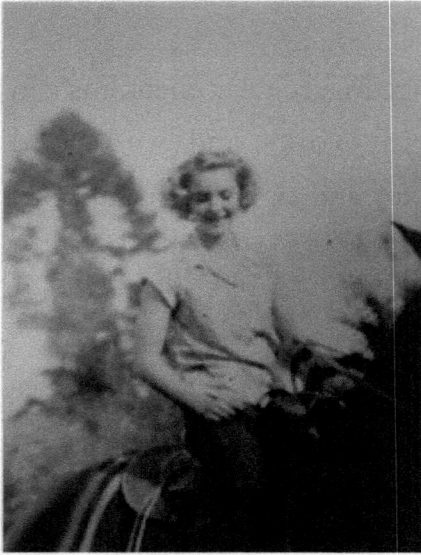

My Mother was one of the most beautiful women in the world, inside and out. Until she wasn't, and the demon alcohol took over her. All the children and other parents in the neighborhood would ask her for advice and private counsel. She kept us unified as a family unit through tremendous struggles.

My Mother went at age fifty-five, November 20, 1988. She didn't learn from drinking herself into alcoholic blackouts. Those voices that told her she wasn't worthy kept her chained to disconnect from her choices to freedom. She let others tell her where her strengths were:

"C'mon Diane. Just one. It's our [whatever the occasion] and it's been years. You got this."

Be mindful of the words you put to the world, inside of you, and outside of you.

She didn't have good emotional or spiritual support from those around her. She had never learned to become her own best friend.

"My Mom signed my Birth Certificate. I was there at the signing of her Death Certificate. My Mom picked out my first outfit, and I chose her last one. My Mom watched me take my first breaths and I watched her take a month of her last."

The Lesson of Forgiveness

The lesson I share with you is this:

If someone in your life hurt you during their addiction, and you're still holding resentment, it will only eat away at *you*.

It's not about them—it's the lack of forgiveness that weighs on your soul, leading you to react in ways that don't align with who you want to be.

Wonder why you're lashing out unexpectedly? That's one sign. There are more.

You won't find peace—the kind that surpasses understanding—until you forgive them *and* yourself.

I didn't realize it was my unresolved resentments that led me to relapse again and again. I couldn't fully learn or meet "me" until it nearly killed me.

You don't have to go that far. I can help guide you to release.

You *can* live your best life. You *don't* have to suffer.

In recovery, we often say suffering is a choice.

My baby sister followed the same path. On her deathbed, barely able to speak, she said, *"I want to live."*

My mother, in her final days, kept repeating, *"I've got it this time. I know I can stay sober and clean this time."*

No one wants to be addicted. No matter what they say when they're drinking or using—trust me.

Healing comes when you let go. You can rise, stay standing, and actually enjoy your time here.

Get a coach, don't do this alone. I wish I had more than just a sponsor. I needed someone to help me *put it all together.*

And it doesn't have to be drugs.

Dis-ease shows up in impulse spending, overeating, or anything that gives instant gratification but leaves you feeling worse.
Those patterns are a sign your *ego* is in control—not your soul.

And one more thing: *You may not have fully grieved someone until you've fully forgiven them.*

Grandma's Final Lesson

My Grandma transitioned in 2000 at age 91, but alcoholism had reared its ugly head at her retirement community. By the time we were called, her apartment was full of alcohol in every possible container. She had Wernicke-Korsakoff syndrome—a condition where alcohol causes the brain to tell you to drink instead of eating—plus creates a dementia that makes your brain forget how to trigger your full swallow reflex. Yep. Feeding tube meals. Alcohol and loneliness at any age can bring on the loss of self.

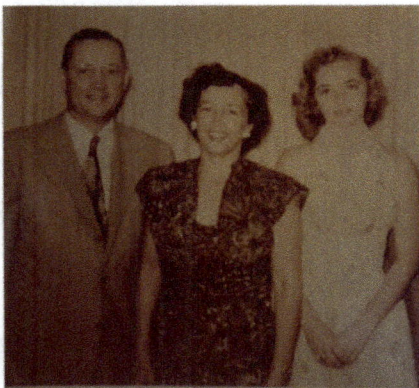

A Few Essential Life Lessons

Mind Your Shadow Voice

Ways to NOT promote the Shadow Voice for yourself or others. Be mindful of what voices you are putting out into the air. They can stick like a catchy commercial that you remember better than your anniversary.

Voices get "stuck" in heads with words like "you can," "everybody should," "that's easy for anyone." If you do not feel as if you measure up, you'll hear that you failed any time the ego can lower your self-worth. Not everyone learns and achieves at the same pace. Be mindful when someone in your circle may not be catching on to something as fast as others. You will be surprised at the friends you will make when you privately offer to help someone. Teach others how to get to know their strengths.

Check in. Care. Share in your journeys.

Without that real-time support, we unintentionally set each other up for something painful. What I call "Shadow Voices in our heads"—those destructive voices that undermine our worth and potential.

The path to resilience is paved with forgiveness, accountability, and the courage to master yourself before life masters you.

Client Results

Here are two examples of results from my commitment to **BE** in the knowing of who I am spiritually and soulfully.

Bruce Gaudette

On October 20, 2019, a pickup truck driver purposefully slammed me and my motorcycle into a guardrail and drove away leaving me for dead. My body sustained massive damage. Physical Therapy helped my body slowly recuperate, but there was an emotional break left untreated..

Elizabeth saw the pain I was in and offered me healing work. I trusted. The massage and coaching she gave me did more than just relax muscles. It healed emotional and spiritual scars. I finally slept for the first time in 5 years. Gratitude is continuing to heal me.

Happy Great Grandpa - D. Strickland

I met this man in AA recovery. He had obvious liver issues and kept saying:

"My grandbabies might have to do without me - I don't see myself living another 10 years. My body hurts too much."

"Dear Coach Elizabeth,

I was 256 lbs.! I am now 203 lbs. I ached all over. Constant physical pain wears you down. My mood is better. Feeling the way I did had me not even wanting to think about living another 10 years. Now, fishing for at least another 20-25 years sounds great, for sure, if I can still feel this great. You taught me I could eat healthily and still enjoy eating. The worst of it. I had to buy new clothes.

Thank you, Elizabeth, for giving me a better life and way of living!

D Strickland. By the way, Coco thanks you too for longer walks every morning."

These stories aren't anomalies. They're evidence.

The Question That Changes Everything

We are all built from genetics, habits, spiritual soul, and created to have choice. We are more than our mistakes, more than our struggles. We are human BEings ~ not just human DOings. Not a cliché. An epiphany. So, when you

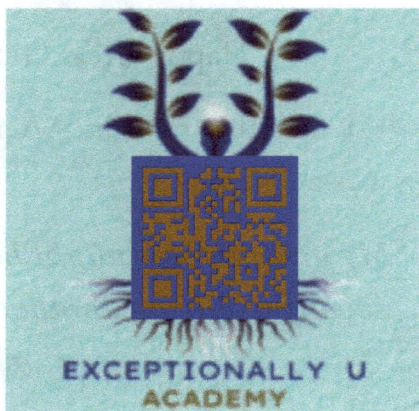

DO, do U well. BE happy, content, confident, and doing what makes you smile.

So, I ask: **Have U Met U?**

Because I believe, without a doubt, you are ready.

Scan to Visit Elizabeth's Website

To begin your own journey, visit FQ3C.com/elizabethv by scanning under the poem below that I wrote for those of you who walked this journey with me, in this chapter.

Elizabeth Villalpando Ellison

CONNECTED BY BIRTH

Born to Belong, The Dance of US

There truly is no reason for lack

When hearts unite, none fall back.

In morning's light, we rise as one,

each day a gift that's just begun.

From egg and sperm, we begin to learn.

Vibrations of voices felt, then heard, not much light.

Our birth from the womb,

our first shared battle.

From cradle's cry to toddler's laugh,

We walk together, half by half.

Your stumbled step becomes my care,

My burden lifted by your prayer.

The schoolyard teaches more than books:

How kindness heals with gentle looks,

How sharing lunch makes spirits bright,

How helping hands make wrongs feel right.

Through youth's bright dreams and middle years,

We hold each other through the tears.

An Apple a Day

Your triumph fills my heart with pride,
My struggles find you by my side.

In golden years when bones grow weak,
The love we've sown is what we reap—
A harvest rich of tender grace,
Reflected in each weathered face.

For nobody demonstrates slack
When love's the thread that keeps us intact.
The joy of waking up is found
In all the ways we come around—

To lift, to hold, to laugh, to mend,
From stranger's nod to dearest friend.
These daily acts of sacred care
Weave golden threads beyond compare.

And when the evening draws us near,
With grateful hearts we hold most dear
The gift of one another's light
That snuggles us to peaceful night.

Elizabeth Villalpando Ellison

From birth's first breath to final rest,

In loving neighbors, we are blessed.

For in this dance of give and take,

We find the joy that souls awake.

About the Author

Elizabeth Villalpando Ellison, graduate of Union Institute & University, Cincinnati, holds a Bachelor of Science in Psychology. Her educational focus on family dynamics, neuroscience, human development, self-awareness, biopsychosocial causes for mood regulation, communication, and didactic well**BE**ing for all age groups has led her to create Exceptionally U Academy.

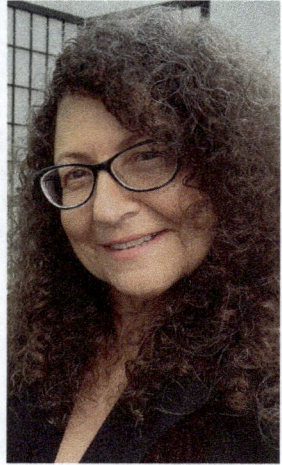

Exceptionally U is being designed as a collaborative structure to bring together a strong and comprehensive opportunity for people of all walks of life to experience "The How To"—how to design mastery with all things that create chaos, depression and anxiety, addictions, suicide prevention, relationships individually or in teams, you name it, she'll help you redesign human disruption into confidence and resilience! Her signature process for mentoring and coaching is called "Have U Met U."

Incorporating "FQ3C" to enhance behavioral baselines, progress tracking with percentile measurement and note archiving HUMU can leverage their client's achievements exponentially. This revolutionary tool is being groomed for use by all demographic groups and industries. You can schedule a demo of her portal by scanning either of the two QR Codes below. You will have identified your design based on your specific needs as fast as their Bot Blinks.

She has helped numerous people with stuttering, sometimes just by talking to them on the phone for 5 minutes and prevented nearly 200 people from committing suicide by talking with and listening to them. She has spoken on numerous stages and at conferences, and she also goes into the streets or canyons to help people who are in crisis.

She's also helped people in recovery programs overcome what she calls "putting down the spoon and picking up the fork"—a metaphor for the shift that often leads to physical health issues, like not fitting into clothes, developing heart or blood sugar problems, or just not being able to move like they used to. She's releasing her e-book this Summer: "How to dance, skip, jump, and run again, and see past your belly!"

Her work spans across Mental Health programs throughout San Diego and the entire far south region of California. She has served as a Project Director for SAMHSA, worked in peer advocacy, and is now working with neurodivergent individuals. She's excited to speak on topics like: Hyperfocus to Hustle.

Elizabeth has also been an Executive Producer with 15 shows weekly on iHeart Radio through Raven International Media. There, she created over 50 podcasts under the brand Home Is Where The Biz Is, which originated during the COVID Pandemic to help guide people with work-from-home ideas and real-life solutions.

Scan To Book a FQ3C demo and experience the magic that occurs when you "see" yourself, right and left brain, values and beliefs. Confident you know what makes you who U are.

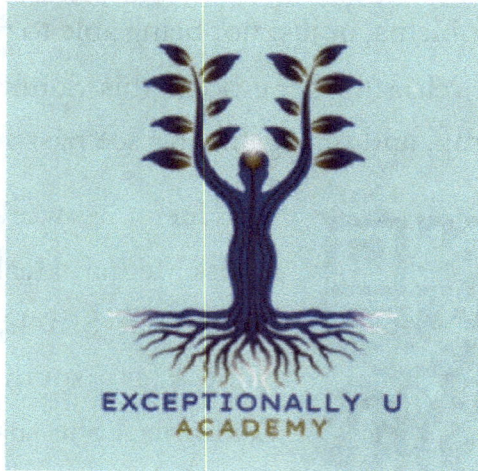

EXCEPTIONALLY U
ACADEMY

HOLISTIC WELLNESS AND FAITH
IN EVERYDAY LIFE

PATRICIA "TRISH' HODGES

CHAPTER SEVEN

HOLISTIC WELLNESS AND FAITH IN EVERYDAY LIFE

Patricia "Trish" Hodges

True wellness is deeper than just physical health. Man is made to walk with a balance of body, soul, and spirit. Each of these intertwined elements work together to shape the way we think, feel, and experience life. The human body is a vessel, carrying us through the world and responding to our environment. The soul— our mind, will, and emotions— guides our thoughts, desires, and relationships. The spirit is our deepest source of inner connection and purpose. Our spirit breathes life and energy into our existence, offering meaning and direction. When all three are synchronized, we create holistic well-being that allows us to thrive in life, not just survive.

By intentionally working toward our well-being, we create a life of joy, vitality, and peace. Let's explore each part of that trinity – Body, Soul, and Spirit. Being informed is the beginning of being transformed!

The Body

It seems today that we are bombarded with how to take care of our physical body. We see ads for exercise equipment, ads for weight loss, ads for supplements which bulk up our muscles and heal our gut... ads, ads everywhere!

We do indeed need to take care of our bodies; however, too many people try to have health "the easy, fast way," which seldom works. We have been given an amazing earthly vessel to walk on this earth. The human body is made with perfected parts, functions, and systems that all work together. When one bone, organ, or valve doesn't do its part, the rest of the body is affected. In spite of possible or real dysfunction in the body, some people have lived in their vessels for over a hundred years.

The body that carries us around each day takes a lot of abuse over the years, so we certainly need to do our best to care for it. Every movement counts in staying healthy. In fact, studies have shown that regular physical exercise can add more than seven years to a person's life.

Physical activity has been proven to balance hormones, improve cardiovascular health, enhance mental health, and improve sleep. It also will boost energy levels so we can practice weight management as well as strengthen our bones and muscles. Exercise will also aid in a healthy mind, and it is well documented that a healthy, positive mindset will help the physical body heal itself. We are thankful for doctors, specialists, and surgeons who help our bodies to be and stay healthy, but we can't rely on them alone. Working on our mindset, exercising regularly, and making use of medicine when needed allows us to create a vibrant future for ourselves.

The Soul

It seems we hear more and more about mental health now, and not just physical wellness. People are seeing counselors, psychologists, and psychiatrists all trying to heal them of past trauma and current fears. Again, just like our bodies, we do need to take care of our soul and perhaps seek professional care. No matter what it takes, we need our soul (mind, will, emotions) to walk in harmony with the rest of our being.

One of the biggest influences in our life is mindset. Mindset is a combination of attitudes, beliefs, and perception. Our mindset will determine how we perceive ourselves, others, events, and life. Numerous studies have shown that mindset will play a gigantic part in our wellness. Have you ever noticed how people who are always looking at the negatives in life are often sick? Many get stuck in a cycle of poor mindset and sickness – then the sickness seems to feed their negative mindset. Getting ourselves out of that negative cycle isn't difficult but requires commitment and focus.

A healthy and strong brain is important, and requires works, just like a healthy and strong physical body. Along with physical exercise which increases oxygen and blood flow to the brain, we need to exercise our brain through reading, creativity, and intentional thoughts. Presenting our brain with new challenges and tasks will help spark receptors in the brain to keep it young and active. However, in today's fast-paced society, we do need to be careful not to overstimulate our brain. Research shows that the brain can only entertain four thoughts (on average) at one time.

Multitasking is necessary at times, but we need to be aware of where our attention is at any given moment. Think of a young single mom who sells real estate. It's dinnertime; she just got off the phone with a finance company, but she needs to find a larger home for a client—tonight. This, while she is cooking (careful, don't burn the casserole!), she is stuffing finance paperwork into an envelope while on the phone, telling her client where they can meet in one hour. When she hangs up with the client, she calls around to find a last-minute babysitter while she feeds her child and helps him with his homework. All the while she is trying to prepare to go make this sale—but wait, she can't go meet this high-dollar client in her exercise wear! No time to shower; she'll do the best she can as she rushes to change, gives instructions to the babysitter, and heads out the door with minutes to spare.

Does that sound familiar? That's no way to operate—short or long-term—and it is no wonder we regularly reach a point of burnout in this era of constant connection. With our minds thinking so much at once, how can a clear thought come through? How can we take care of others when we don't take care of ourselves? We must learn to "practice hitting pause" at some point each day. Just to sit, close our eyes and begin to allow peace to pour into ourselves. Even if your only private moment is in your bathroom – pause. Of course, a nice walk in the neighborhood or sitting in our yard, letting the sun bathe down upon us, would be ideal. There is so much power in stillness that it is more a matter of doing it rather than focusing on where to pause. Don't allow perfect to be the enemy of done—find a way to pause daily!

Keeping positive thoughts is key to holistic wellness. With positive pathways, we can tap into the brain's ability to create inner peace. However, negative thoughts can quietly intrude into our mind, shaping our thoughts and actions in a destructive way. One thing we need to be careful of is not generalize or using exclusionary language like "I never win" or "I always lose." Focus on what is true, not on assumptions or generalizations. We need to be aware of thinking we can read someone else's mind. Only they really know what is going on in their head, and we can only control ourselves. Our mind can work to stay positive as we change those old patterns of thinking.

The well-known neuroscientist, Dr. Carolyn Leaf, has been working on the mind-brain connection for over four decades. She was one of the first to study how the brain is wired – and rewired. She explains how neural pathways have been created in the brain when people suffer trauma. These traumatic pathways become our negative thought patterns over time. Dr. Leaf shows that we can build new neural pathways, just like creating a new path in your yard. Rewiring our minds to think in broader terms than only negative takes time and conscious effort but is worth the investment.

As you travel to one part of your yard, perhaps to the trash can or a garage, you will see the development of a path over time; a place where grass doesn't grow because you walk on it all the time. That's like the pathways in our brain. We can either allow the negative pathways to continue making a deeper, wider path or intentionally change the way we think for the better. If we intentionally focus on positive thoughts, new neural pathways will be created and replace the negative pathways, based on our intentional thinking. Let's make that the pathway which is more often travelled.

Other scientific studies have proven that an optimistic, grateful attitude, can decrease the likelihood of heart attacks and strokes by over thirty percent. Other studies show less depression and less anxiety in those who have a grateful and forgiving life. There is obviously a connection between our mind, our physical body, and the importance of thinking positive thoughts.

When negative thought patterns arise, you can choose to reroute them to positive ones. One way to reroute a negative thought to refocused uplifting thoughts is to take three slow deep breaths. Take time to focus on your breathing – inhale slowly through your nose, then exhale slowly through your mouth. This way, you can help stop the negative thought as it is happening. This helps calm your fight or flight reflex, which allows for you to better control your thoughts."

Another trick to avoid those negative thoughts is to make a list of positive possibilities or outcomes prior to a known stressor, a list you can pull out to read and refocus when negativity arises. A list of positive affirmations to use in general can help to redirect self-doubt. For centuries, philosophers and spiritual teachers have proclaimed that "you are what you think," and we see modern psychology using Cognitive Behavior Therapy (CBT) in a similar way to help refocus negative thought patterns with techniques to help us think differently.

Emotions can also cause negative thoughts if allowed. An interesting fact I heard years ago, and again just recently, is that an emotion or feeling only lasts for ninety seconds. Ninety seconds! So why do we stay angry all day or pout for two weeks? Our thoughts! Negative thoughts will cause those emotions to rise up and work against us if we allow them. Positive thinking can silence those emotions. If you find yourself walking in a negative emotion, stop and intentionally refocus the thoughts carrying you to that emotion. Breathe and take the other path. As we practice moving into quieter focus, we will see that our mind no longer hears the noises of life. In quietness we are able to think more clearly and relax. It is important to remember that positive thinking is more than a mindset — it is a tool for transformation.

As we grow in gratitude, mindfulness, and positive thought patterns, we will see our life shaping into something beautiful. We begin to capture the beauty around us and in others. Our brain is full of dynamic power; using it properly, we can see life as full of astounding opportunities—and surprisingly fulfilling.

Spirit

Positive thinking and spirituality are distinct, and yet astonishingly intertwined. A heart full of optimism and gratitude enhances spiritual well-being, just as faith, prayer, and meditation cultivate inner peace and joy within the soul. None of us is perfect, and we all have room to grow, but at least nurturing all three areas gives us a better outlook. It's important to realize that the human body, soul, and spirit were created to work together in harmony. The spirit of a human is the innermost part, the essence of who we are and what we become. Our spirit was created to connect with the creator of all heaven and earth. God created man with a body to function and do things. He gave man a mind so that he could think and do things. He also gave man a spirit to equip him to do things. Seems like there's a common thread between all these; we get to "do things" in life. Ephesians 2:10 says, "For we are God's handiwork, created in Christ Jesus to do good works, which God prepared in advance for us to do."

We are God's creation with each of us gifted to do good. God's plan was for man to walk with God's Spirit; for the Spirit to dwell within him. Because of rebellion in the garden of Eden, that intimate relationship between Adam, Eve, and God was severed. Much of what we see going on in the world today is not necessarily good. Murder, suicide, and depression have reached all-time highs. The further we are from the Fall, the more sin creeps into this world. Awareness of the body, soul, and spirit connection is needed, perhaps now more than ever.

God created man to be in fellowship with Him, to be connected with Him forever. It is not God's will that any human should perish or be separated from His love. Consequently, in His ultimate wisdom, a plan of reconciliation brought us back into relationship through Jesus Christ. Within this reconciled state, man receives new life. That new life comes when our spirit is enlivened by God's

Spirit. I've heard an analogy of this new life in relation to jump-starting a dead car battery. The life (energy) from a good battery sparks the old battery to function once again. The Holy Spirit sparks our spirits so that we are emboldened to be the person we were created to be. Don't squander your spark!

Ancient practices such as meditation, prayer, and communal gatherings are gaining recognition for their combined psychological, physiological, and spiritual benefits. The blending of the spiritual legacies of the past with the practical challenges of the present promotes a future in which wellness is as much about spiritual harmony as it is about physical and mental health. The Bible is a fantastic foundation to living in wholeness. Scripture offers profound insights into living a life filled with positivity and purpose.

The Bible encourages reflection on the positive: "Finally, brethren, whatever things are true, whatever things are noble, whatever things are just, whatever things are pure, whatever things are lovely, whatever things are of good report, if there is any virtue and if there is anything praiseworthy—meditate on these things" (Philippians 4:8.) An ancient verse, from Proverbs 17:22, reminds us that, "A merry heart does good, like medicine, but a broken spirit dries the bones." Embracing this cheerful heart catalyzes holistic wellness – body, soul, and spirit. Even cancer doctors prescribe watching comedy shows to lead their patients to laughter. That laughter, in turn, will help the physical body heal faster, and the heavy load on the mind will be lightened. Laughter is amazing for holistic well-being. Think about it… it's nearly impossible to be angry with someone when you are laughing with them. When laughing, our brain and emotions begin to run in the direction of joy, as our body heals itself.

Hope led by faith causes greater resilience and emotional health, which will foster patience, love, and understanding of ourselves and others. Each of these is an essential quality that deepen human relationships. In the ever-changing landscape of wellness and personal growth, the union of right thinking and faith will offer great transformative potential. Faith greatly influences interpersonal relationships as gratitude and optimism enhance our well-being. Communities rooted in faith often show increased emotional support, reinforcing that we thrive when we lift each other up.

With this optimistic faith, we will launch towards a fruitful life, focused on our true purpose. Purpose! We each have a purpose in life. Think of visionaries like Martin Luther King Jr. and Mahatma Gandhi. They were driven by faith to fight for justice. Mother Teresa demonstrated how unwavering faith developed compassion, love, and service to others. Her service to mankind led to many lasting community improvements. Corrie Ten Boom, who survived four months in a WWII concentration camp, often shared her favorite poem. This poem, written by Grant Tullar, describes how life may look like a mess, but it creates a beautiful picture.

Life is But a Weaving

My life is but a weaving between my God and me.

I cannot choose the colors He weaveth steadily.

Oft' times He weaveth sorrow; and I in foolish pride

Forget He sees the upper and I the underside.

Not 'til the loom is silent and the shuttles cease to fly

Will God unroll the canvas and reveal the reason why.

The dark threads are as needful in the weaver's skillful hand

As the threads of gold and silver in the pattern He has planned.

He knows, He loves, He cares; nothing this truth can dim.

He gives the very best to those who leave the choice to Him.

This poet understood a joyous outlook on life. Looking at a tapestry on one side, we see a multitude of colors, intricate patterns creating an intentional masterpiece of art. Through the ages, each thread has been placed specifically to tell a story of triumph, love, family, and wealth. However, if we look at the backside of the beautiful piece of artwork, we see a chaotic mess of knots, tangles, and strands. Quite different from the front of the tapestry, the work we see on the other side appears disorderly and unfinished. This look at the back of the tapestry is much like moments in our life when we can't see the entire picture, or a positive outcome.

But just as an artist weaves the colorful strands of thread into a thing of beauty, every trial we face in life becomes part of a greater design to be seen at a later time. The Bible, in Jeremiah 29:11, tells us that God has a good, beautiful "tapestry" for each of us, saying, "For I know the thoughts that I think toward you, says the Lord, thoughts of peace and not of evil, to give you a future and a hope." So, God's plan for us is good, and He created us with the ability to fulfill that plan. Ephesians 2:10 states, "For we are His workmanship, created in Christ Jesus for good works, which God prepared beforehand that we should walk in them." We are not a puppet, but a free agent who yields to the knowledge and faithfulness of our Creator. Only He knows what the best direction for our life is, and only He knows how to make our life beautiful.

Just as our ideal weight or high IQ are not destinations, faith is not a destination; we have an adventurous journey ahead, nurturing each of us. We can create a path toward a life of wellness when we ponder the Word of God, stand in steadfast hope, and prayer. Quieting the noise of life and sin around us can become a daily routine to mental and spiritual enrichment. Gratitude, hope, and purpose fuse together to enrich our wellness.

Personal Testimony

Having an optimistic faith is key to human wholeness, but I admit I have not always walked in it. It has been over the years that I have learned to surrender fear, pain and uncertainty to God. I have learned to expect the best out of every situation. I have determined that if I'm not seeing the "best," I know God is not done yet with the situation.

My childhood was filled with health struggles, and my teenage years were marked by trauma. To drown out the pain, I turned to drugs and alcohol. They were temporary painkillers, but I eventually found myself in utter hopelessness and alone. My body was filled with disease, my mind only looked at the past, at what others had done to me, and at my own mistakes. As my mind continued to create deep paths of negativity, my spirit was especially in a coma. If you have ever been at this point, then you understand what it was like to live with no hope.

One day, after crying out in despair, I felt led to open the nightstand drawer beside my bed. Inside, I found The Living Bible that had been given to me years prior. I kept it close by but never opened it to a single page. As I sat on the edges of my bed to read, I discovered something life changing. I discovered that God is real, and I was made for a purpose. That statement boggled my mind.

After days of reading this new book, I began to realize there was a future that I could look forward to. I surrendered to the idea that I could think more healing thoughts and that God had a plan for my life—a plan to prosper instead of suffer. Instead of listening to the negative inner voices, trying to condemn me, I chose to dwell on the positive. My trek in life has never been the same since the day I surrendered negativity. My focus of despair was shifted to one of empowerment, rewiring my thoughts towards a pathway of possibility and healing."

I am now privileged to lead other women to God's saving grace and a total life change. Many have come to me in despair, as I knew all too well. Realizing Jesus had bought their freedom, they begin to think differently and walk in hope. They began to say positive things about themselves and others, as well as becoming part of a positive mindset community. What a wonderful marriage of faith and optimism. As well as soul and spirit wellness, I have seen many of these women overcome health issues they've had for years. The synchronicity of their body, soul and spirit is a testament to the marvels of creation.

Your Time to Shine

An optimistic faith offers stability amid life's uncertainties. Faith and a positive mindset do not promise a life free from hardships, but I have found that standing in faith enables us to weather any storm. At a time when life takes a sudden turn; when we become unemployed, or a doctor gives us a grave diagnosis, a positive mindset will help us make clear, wise decisions. Faith is our anchor in hope, so we can chase the vision of God's good plan for us. The storm may not be pleasant, but we will always weather it. Faith says to cast "all your care upon Him; for He (God) cares for you." (I Peter 5:7).

I am an advocate of daily affirmations. Scientific research supports that daily declarations of positive affirmations can lower stress hormone levels, boost self-esteem, strength, and resilience. Faith functions similarly, providing emotional stability and guiding individuals through challenges with hope. Here are a few I like to say to remind myself that I can "do life" with a smile:

Today I choose joy, peace, and gratitude because each moment is a gift

I am strong, capable, and equipped to handle whatever comes my way

I am fearfully and wonderfully made with a purpose for my life

God sustains me and guides my steps; I choose to walk in His good plan

I radiate positivity, hope, and encouragement to those around me

I can testify that intentionally keeping truth (positive thoughts, the Word of God) in the forefront on my mind allows me to experience peace beyond anyone's understanding—and you can, too. As faith and positive thinking intertwine with our daily life, we can experience stability, healing, and hope in the most challenging times and circumstances. By merging Bible, science, and experience, you cultivate a holistic approach to wellness. To craft our most fulfilled life, we need to nurture our precious body, soul, and spirit.

Honor your body with rest, healthy choices, and moments of quiet. Honor your soul with joy and pursuing purpose. Allow yourself grace through life's difficult times. The essence of who you are, your spirit, is strengthened when you connect with faith, love, and a purpose greater than yourself.

It's time for you to lift your head up, put your shoulders back, and walk into new wholeness. With your renewed, faith-filled mindset, you will begin to see changes – not only in your body, but also in your situations. You will begin to see favor at your employment, a widening supportive circle, and much more as you launch into your future.

I encourage you to seek healing, strive for inner growth, and let faith be your anchor. Wholeness is a matter of balance. It's intentionally choosing each day to feed your entire being with what lifts and sustains you. With faith and hope, you will be propelled and guided into a new, more confident, healthier you.

Being mindful and living in alignment with body, soul, and spirit, life will become more meaningful, richer, and full of calm. You were created to be rich in peace, strength, wisdom, and divine purpose. Wholeness doesn't come easy; it's something you need to go after with all your might. It takes a hunger and determination to have a healthy body, a peaceful soul, and a strong spirit. The venture is well worth it! With holistic wellness, you will be on a transformational journey, and you will watch your life unfold like a beautiful spring flower.

"The blending of the spiritual legacies of the past with the practical challenges of the present promotes a future in which wellness is as much about spiritual harmony as it is about physical and mental health."

About the Author

With a deep commitment to marrying a positive mindset and faith, Patricia "Trish" Hodges is dedicated to illuminating paths toward transformative lives. As an author, course creator, and spiritual director, her journey has been defined by a passion for guiding others to discover their full potential. Through her works, she inspires individuals to embrace the best they can be – Body, Soul, & Spirit.

With a background in teaching, psychology, and Bible, Trish weaves positive psychology principles with spiritual insight. Her approach offers a unique perspective that resonates with those seeking deeper meaning and purpose in life. She strives to create a supportive, safe space for growth, empowering women to live with intention and faith at the forefront of their journey.

Contact Patricia

Links: Facebook @ LOOKING UP 24 / Trish Hodges
https://www.facebook.com/profile.php?id=6157152038043

Linkedin @ Patricia 'Trish' Hodges
https://www.linkedin.com/in/patricia-trish-hodges-6b9a134a/

Website: https://www.lookingup24.org

You Tube @ LOVING LIFE HOPE / Trish Hodges
https://www.youtube.com/@LovingLifeHope

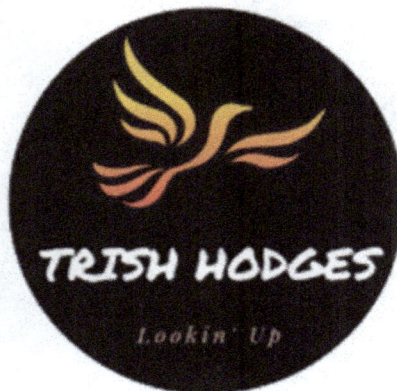

THE UNORTHODOX PRESCRIPTION

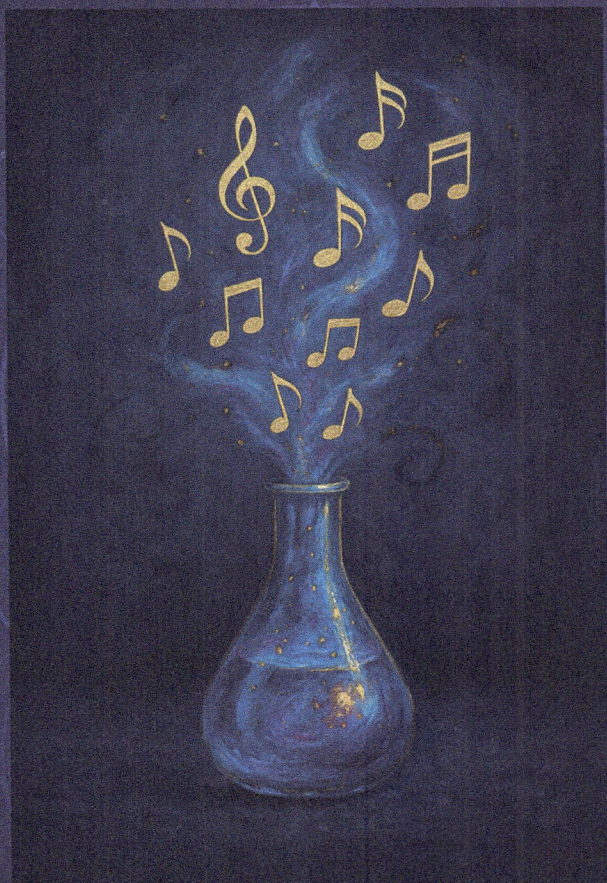

SueZee Finley

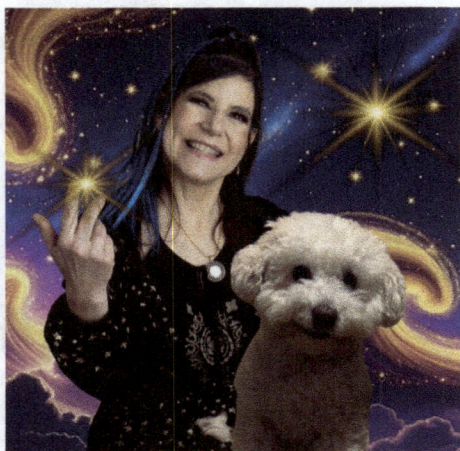

To my Puffball Taji,

My fluffy sidekick, my little sorceress in training.

Though I can't hold you in my arms,

I feel you in the music,

in the stillness between notes,

in the quiet knowing of my heart.

I know you're out there—

dancing through the stars,

tail wagging, paws waving,

getting all the belly rubs from angels,

utterly smitten from the first tail wag—how could they
not be?

Your love lives on in every healing, every laugh,

every moment I remember who I am.

You were, and still are, my magic.

CHAPTER EIGHT

THE UNORTHODOX PRESCRIPTION

SueZee Finley

We've all heard the adage 'An apple a day keeps the doctor away,' and been told to eat our veggies. However, have you ever heard that frequencies are nutrients, capable of restoring vibrant health faster than any pharmaceutical drug on the market? I certainly hadn't – until the night my body staged a full-scale rebellion. This unexpected revolt set me on a transformative healing journey, one that allowed me to ditch my side-effect-laden prescriptions, reclaim my health, and ignite a never-ending passion for the restorative power of sound, frequency, and color.

It seemed to come out of nowhere. One night, I went to bed, and three hours later, I jolted awake in a blaze of pain so intense and surreal that I was convinced I must be trapped in a nightmare, but I wasn't. I was fully awake!

When I tried to sit up, my stomach wouldn't move – more unbearable pain. It felt as if there was a tight band choking my waist, an undefinable crushing force literally squeezing the breath out of me. As I tried bending my knees, a burning, piercing pain shot through my body. When I tried pushing myself up with my hands, it felt like my body had turned into a block of stone; my body was locked down. It was as if each of my joints had been doused in crazy glue and they were now immovable. And whichever part of my body I attempted to move felt like it was on fire.

For the next few hours, the pain rendered me breathless. As I rocked back and forth in agony, I visualized that the crazy glue preventing my every single movement was cracking and falling away, allowing my joints to open. When I was able to finally rock myself up to sit, I wanted to call for help; I had been home alone through all of this. However, my fingers were so swollen it was almost impossible to dial the phone. It was so hard to lift, the phone felt like it was 500 pounds. It took 30 minutes to dial and talk to my sister. Janet and her husband Joe immediately came to my rescue. They literally had to carry me out of the house to the ER.

As they carried me out, I had a flashback to a couple of years prior, when I was diagnosed with Lupus and Sjögren's. At that time, the doctor advised that as long as I didn't get stressed, I would be fine. Really? Who doesn't get stressed?

Although, I had more stress than I cared to admit. I had been the primary caregiver for three terminally ill family members shortly after going through a divorce. However, my body's current reaction seemed extremely harsh.

Broken and In Agony

The doctor told me that my body was experiencing an extreme Lupus flare and I needed to be put on a megadose of Prednisone immediately, to stop any further damage.

I was in so much pain, I don't remember the doctor giving me any encouraging words before I left. I went home believing that this was a permanent condition.

As I lay on my couch, which was all I could do, I wondered how I would be able to care for myself. Would I have to get rid of my dog and three cats? Who would care for my frail, ailing sister Joanne and her fragile little dog? I was in shock, disoriented, with no idea what was going on or what to do next.

Before all this, my sister Joanne had two nicknames for me: 'Energizer Bunny SueZee' and 'Pack Horse SueZee' because I took care of everyone and buzzed around happily doing so. But now, I felt like someone had ripped my batteries out. As I lay there like a broken toy, I wondered what my future held.

Roller–coaster Ride of Hope

Fifteen hours later, a miracle happened! The swelling was down, and the pain was fading away! "Woohoo, I'm cured!" I thought. For a week, I felt great! When I went back to my doctor for a follow-up visit, feeling like a bouncing ray of sunshine, he literally eclipsed my light. "This is not a miracle, SueZee, it was the megadose of prednisone that did this," he said. He informed me that if I wanted to continue to feel like this, then I would have to take immunosuppressors for the rest of my life.

He continued, "Your immune system is breaking down faster than it can repair itself." To drive the point deeper, he added, "Your body is attacking itself and your cells are eating each other." As he said this, my mind conjured up the image of Pac-Man running around munching on my cells, and my heart sank.

"Nooo!" I screamed inside my head. "I don't even take an aspirin, and now this? No, there has to be another option," I blurted out to him. He explained that this was my only option. With a prescription in hand, I went home feeling utterly defeated and betrayed by my body. I was devastatingly sad about the thought of taking immunosuppressors for the rest of my life. It seemed absurd, deliberately wrecking what I'd spent my life building. He also told me that with Lupus, I had to stay out of the sun, no weightlifting or martial arts, which

I did regularly to stay healthy. He said my body needed to reserve as much energy as possible to stop it from breaking down.

Scared and feeling hopeless, I contemplated taking the immunosuppressors because he said it could give me a relatively normal life. However, once home, I did what all doctors tell you not to do... I read the package insert which listed all the 'possible' side effects. I immediately called my doctor and made another appointment. At his office, we had this turning point conversation: "I'm concerned about taking these pills."

"Why?" he asked.

"The side effects include blindness," I said as I hit my finger on the line that stated this on the insert.

His casual response still echoes in my memory: "That almost rarely never happens!" What does that even mean? Think about that – would you fly on a plane if the pilot said, "Welcome to Almost Airlines, we almost rarely never crash!"?

Standing Up for Me

So, you guessed it – I left his office that day and never returned. I was 51 years old and scared about what my future held. I was told I would need to go on disability because my health would continue to go downhill, especially since I chose not to take immunosuppressors. However, this marked the beginning of my journey into the unknown world of alternative healing, which later led me to my passion for sound therapy.

As weeks went by, it seemed my body was indeed declining like he said. My body grew stiffer, pain crept in, and I felt weak and exhausted. I was experimenting with many different alternative treatments. Luckily, I was introduced to a great naturopathic doctor whom I started seeing immediately. I was also blessed to have amazing chiropractors and acupuncturists. I eliminated known inflammatory triggers: gluten, sugar, and all processed foods. My naturopath recommended a rigorous supplement protocol, along with tiny, highly nutritious, organic meals, which I faithfully followed. It gradually addressed my body's underlying imbalances. The inflammation receded enough that I was able to walk again – a huge victory! But one that still felt somewhat hollow.

Wake Up Call

My former energy levels seemed forever out of reach. My once vibrant life shrunk to only three hours of daily functionality, punctuated with afternoon naps and marathon nighttime sleep sessions. The most devastating to me was the thick mental fog that hovered over my head, smothering my creativity, curiosity, and innovative spirit – qualities that once defined my essence and made my life magical.

The funny thing is, I was so thrilled just to be walking again that I didn't fully grasp how limited my life had become until someone asked me out on a date. Reflecting on that conversation now, it feels like a scene ripped straight from a painfully awkward romantic comedy.

The poor guy made the fatal mistake of starting with an innocent question: "What do you like to eat?" Without missing a beat, I launched into an overly detailed explanation of my strict diet of tiny meals consisting of only organic, grass-fed meat and vegetables. I explained how my body was too fragile to digest large portions and how everything had to be timed perfectly with my supplements. His eyes rolled slightly, but he pressed on.

"Okay… so, how about the beach?" he asked, still hopeful. That's when I hit him with an unsolicited TED Talk on lupus and photosensitivity. I vividly described how sunlight triggered flares, likening myself to the 'Invisible Man' – hat, sunglasses, long sleeves, gloves, the whole ensemble. "That's me at the beach," I declared triumphantly. The guy blinked but didn't retreat.

Undeterred (and unfortunately, neither did I stop talking), he suggested going to the movies. "Oh, no can do," I replied.

"I need to be in bed by 9 p.m., or my body crashes." It was much later, thanks to my brain fog, that I realized he was asking me out on a date. Feeling guilty for shutting him down every turn, I agreed to a 7 p.m. movie; where I promptly fell asleep by 7:15. Had popcorn been allowed in my diet and sitting in my lap, I might have face-planted in it.

Needless to say, I didn't go out on any more dates.

That was my wake-up call. I had not realized how ridiculously complicated my life had become. Some days I couldn't get out of bed, and when I did, I could barely stay awake. I missed most social functions. My life was unrecognizable to what it once had been. No more sculpting, yoga, and martial arts. Obviously, no dating. As it was, I had put all these things on hold for years to be a caregiver and now that my caregiving duties were over, I felt weak and useless.

The timing of it all felt especially harsh, so I vented my frustrations to my doctor about wanting more out of life. His response was blunt: "You're lucky to be walking at all without immunosuppressors. Returning to your former vitality? Highly unlikely."

As if that wasn't enough to crush my spirit, when I got home that day after the doctor's visit, I turned on the TV only to hear Dr. Wayne Dyer's voice booming: "Don't die with your music still inside you!" That was it! I broke down sobbing. My music? My magic? Gone. Or so I thought…

Staying Open

Luckily, true magic has a way of finding its way back, and fate intervened during a weekend trip to New Paltz, NY, where my friend Marla convinced me to attend an alternative health convention with her. Despite my reservations, something, perhaps destiny, pulled me forward.

The convention was everything I dreamed it would be! I listened to lectures from leading alternative healing practitioners from around the world. On breaks, we curiously roamed the vendors' area filled with everything you could possibly think of on natural healing: books, crystals, tuning forks, and exotic healing practitioners. I was beyond excited. I felt almost normal for a precious hour as I explored the plethora of offerings with genuine curiosity.

Then, without warning, exhaustion hit me like kryptonite hits Superman. A cold sweat beaded on my skin, and my knees began to go weak. My heart started to race as I frantically scanned the area for a place to sit before I fell down. I felt like I was going to black out at any moment, and then I spotted him as he spotted me — the sound therapist who was smiling and waving me over. I got there as fast as I could, dragging my legs that seemed to weigh two tons each.

When I sat down, I took the name badge off over my head (I don't know why I thought it would make me feel lighter) as I plopped onto the chair. This mysterious man smoothly floated a microphone into my hands. His motion seemed oddly graceful, magical, and surreal. I vaguely registered his instructions to speak into it and did. Then he helped me onto the massage table, sliding headphones onto my ears, placing a lavender-scented mask over my eyes, and wrapping me in a cozy fleece blanket.

I still get chills thinking about what happened next. Within seconds, I felt swept away as otherworldly sounds pulsed through both the headphones and the table. I experienced what felt like an internal symphony. Golden lights and stars danced behind my closed eyes as vibrations awakened every cell in my body. It felt like my cells were singing in delight as negative thoughts rose like soap bubbles and dissolved into the ethereal soundscape. My shoulders, which held permanent residence close to my ears from all the stress I endured over the years, were gently swept down by a wave of sound that coursed through me from head to toe, lowering my shoulders and wrapping me in this blanket of peace, tranquility, and bliss.

I fell into the deepest sleep I had experienced in years. When Greg, the practitioner, gently tapped my shoulder, I heard a whisper in my ears, a message that filled me with joy, but I lost the words as my eyes popped open. It was as if I'd awakened into a new dimension of vitality. My mind sparkled with a clarity I hadn't known in decades. "What just happened?" I exclaimed, my voice ringing with newfound energy.

"Your voice is the composite of all your body's frequencies. I analyzed them and played back exactly what you needed. Think of frequencies as nutrients – I just fed your body the music it needed." Greg's profound words shifted my inner thoughts, connecting with my deep knowing and wisdom. He then handed me two CDs and a printout: a personalized list of harmonious items that vibrated in my frequency, including emerald stones, green clothing, specific essential oils, and music in the notes of 'C' and 'G', all carefully chosen to restore my energetic balance.

My 'Frequency Party' Prescription

I remember joking to myself, "Is this a prescription to go shopping?" Best prescription ever! What girl doesn't want an excuse to buy colorful clothes, gemstones, and fragrant oils!! Super bonus, I was in the most extraordinary vendors' room I had ever seen! This was my permission slip to buy everything I needed (something a lot of us hold back on, since most caregivers put everyone else's needs above their own), but not today! It was a shopping spree just for me!

The vendors' area that had felt overwhelming and hard to navigate just 30 minutes earlier now seemed like a walk in the park – no, the candy store. I felt like a kid on a magical treasure hunt, with my newfound energy and joy propelling me forward. With my unusual prescription in hand, I began my hunt. The first thing that resonated in me was the most beautiful sounds coming from across the room – a man playing a hand-hammered and engraved brass Himalayan singing bowl. I had always wanted one, and it turned out to be in the note that I needed: 'G'. Taking this as a sign, I purchased it immediately.

It was huge, bigger than a giant salad bowl you have at large family gatherings. He didn't have a bag large enough and offered to hold the singing bowl behind his table until the end of the day; however, with my newfound strength, I insisted on carrying it. I was so enamored with it, I wanted to hold it all day. The vendor loved my enthusiasm; he laughed and plopped a red velvet pouch containing two tuning forks as a gift and winked, "I know you are going to love these too."

My treasure hunt continued as I circled the room. A beautiful hand-painted green silk scarf caught my eye – perfect, as green was one of my prescribed colors. I had the vendor drop it into the bowl. At the essential oils' booth, I found both scents I needed: peppermint and cedarwood. Each item went into my singing bowl. I felt like a kid trick-or-treating, but instead of getting candy, my bowl was becoming a vessel of healing treasures. The final item on my list was an emerald, and remarkably, I found a vendor selling raw, uncut emerald stones.

A New Life

Looking into my singing bowl of collected treasures: the emerald, two tuning forks, essential oils, and the green scarf, I felt an amazing energy as I was struck by a lightning bolt of clarity: I wanted to become a sound therapist. I wanted everyone to experience the profound healing I had just experienced. I wanted to write prescriptions for music, color, essential oils, and gemstones. Most importantly, I wanted everyone to know about an alternative to harmful prescription drugs, a natural and most delightful one! One with side effects that result in peace, joy, and energy.

If that wasn't exciting enough, another amazing effect that surprised me in the most wonderful way was my newfound ability to manifest things. I didn't fully understand this mysterious phenomenon until I took a class with Jonathan Goldman (a master in sound healing and harmonics with over fifty years' experience). He revealed his secret formula: Intention + Vibration = Manifestation. I can attest that this method works amazingly well.

Within a week of returning home, I received a check from my insurance company that allowed me to purchase the acoustic sound table and voice frequency scan equipment that had given me my life back. I secured my dream office and named my practice Acoustic Therapeutix. Plus, I was accepted into a three-year sound therapy degree program at a fantastic school.

This ignited a deep passion to continue delving into this amazing field with its infinite depth, more amazing than anything I had experienced in my life. It gave me such joy; it was an instrumental part of my healing. With each sound therapy class, I was filled with the greatest awe.

During my first three years of learning, I immersed myself in sacred geometry, color therapy, light therapy, tuning forks, singing bowls, toning, humming, and drumming. With each class, my excitement grew. I couldn't help but wonder: How had I gone so long without knowing this whole field existed? How had I not known that everything is frequency and that we are all electrical, light, and magnetic beings?

I went from having no energy, clarity or focus to having an amazing new, awe-inspiring career as a sound therapist, where each and every day I learned something new. It's never-ending excitement discovering all the ways that the frequencies from sound, color, gemstones, along with what we get from each other, can completely recharge our cells and restore us. Sometimes I feel I need to pinch myself to make sure that all this is real. We live in an awesome, magical universe.

Amazing Mentors

I have been blessed with amazing teachers, and it has been an honor to learn from them.

I will always remember my very first voice class with Vickie Dodd (a pioneer in sound and body work). Her opening statement left me speechless: "Of all the tools in your sound healing toolbox, your voice is the most important." My jaw dropped. Partly because I had just invested a small fortune in acoustic sound equipment (which I still cherish), but mostly because I had been completely unaware that my own voice was perhaps the most powerful healing instrument of all. What she taught was so simple and accessible for everyone to have immediate, tangible results.

Vickie introduced me to the remarkable power of the 'hum'. Despite my substantial investment in sophisticated acoustic equipment, I was thrilled to learn how something so fundamentally simple as our 'hum' could create such profound effects.

The science behind this is fascinating. Researchers discovered that humming generates nitric oxide – a natural vasodilator that relaxes our cardiovascular system and lowers blood pressure. It simultaneously stimulates the vagus nerve, dramatically reducing stress levels, while exhibiting impressive anti-bacterial, anti-viral, and anti-fungal properties. A simple hum contains all this healing potential!

This knowledge proved invaluable during the COVID pandemic, during which I pivoted to conducting online workshops. The humming exercise quickly became my signature activity. During one hysterically memorable session, I forgot to start my timer and inadvertently had the group humming for over fifteen minutes. This particular technique requires participants to place their fingers over their eyes and thumbs over their ears to create a sensory cocoon. When I finally realized we had gone well beyond our usual time, I discreetly peeked through my fingers only to discover everyone staring back at me, their eyes laughing with tears through their peek-a-boo fingers.

What followed was silly, contagious laughter. If anyone had walked in, they would have thought we were all stoned. We had all entered such an amazing state of bliss that none of us could stop. The laughter rippled through our screens, connecting us in different parts of the world, despite our physical separation. A testament to how something as simple as a collective hum could transcend barriers and create a moment of pure joy. The next day, my Facebook was swarming with bee emojis, and I was crowned the 'Queen Bee of Happiness.' That's how the 'Happiness Hive Group' was formed, and later my 'Happiness Now Network App & Podcast.'

We are Electrical Beings

The deeper I explored sound therapy, the more I understood a profound truth: we're not just biochemical beings; we are electric, magnetic, and light. The statement that wrapped it all up in a bow for me came from mentor Dr. John Beaulieu (one of the foremost philosophers and major innovators in sound healing therapies). He told a story from a talk to medical students who questioned him about the existence of energy fields and chakras. The students said they didn't see chakras in the cadavers they were working on. He responded, "Of course you wouldn't – the bodies are dead, their energy and life force have already left."

Lightning bolt moment! Everything made sense to me from that day forward. When he taught us how to use tuning forks, the results were astonishing. Every person affects another. It's a chain reaction of happiness that I love setting off! Today, I don't leave home without my tuning forks. I tune people wherever I go! I am eternally grateful to Dr. Beaulieu for his amazing work and for the generosity with which he shares it!!

The Magnificent Symphony

In 500 BC, when Greek philosopher Pythagoras declared rocks to be 'frozen music', he wasn't merely indulging in poetic fancy. His intuitive understanding, now validated by modern scientific research reveals the truth about our world: every element of nature is engaged in a constant, harmonious song. From the gentle swaying of grass blades to the vibrant hues of blooming flowers, from the towering majesty of trees to the very ground beneath our feet, all of creation resonates with its own unique frequency. This universal concert of vibrations creates an intricate tapestry of sound, imperceptible to our ears but felt deeply in our cells. This is why nature is so harmonizing and uplifting to our mind, body, and soul.

The first sound healing session changed the way I see and experience everything. I have a sense of connection and knowing that gives my life flow and ease.

In the end, my journey taught me that true healing isn't about fighting against illness; it's about harmonizing the body, it's about tuning into the magnificent symphony that's always playing within and around us. Every morning when I wake up, I no longer see a body that betrayed me, but rather an instrument waiting to be played in perfect harmony with the world, and when it's a little off, I simply tune it!

Remember: "You have the power to write your own frequency prescription." Nature has already embedded within you and around you every note, every rhythm, every healing vibration you'll ever need – you are both the composer and conductor of your magnificent symphony. Your heart knows the melody of your highest healing, your soul carries the rhythm of your deepest wisdom, and your spirit holds the key to every frequency that will restore your harmony. So go ahead – put on that colorful scarf, breathe in that uplifting essential oil, and let your voice sing your soul into bliss. "Your symphony isn't just waiting to begin – it's already playing within you, waiting for you to pick up the conductor's wand and lead the orchestra of your own extraordinary life."

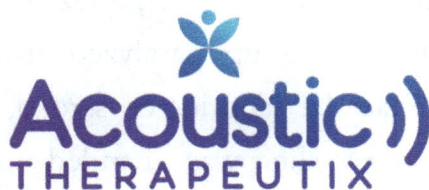

Acoustic))
THERAPEUTIX

About the Author

Meet SueZee Finley – The Sound Sorceress of Freedom and Joy

A visionary guide, teacher of vibrational healing, and creator of soul-shifting experiences, SueZee invites you on a journey where sound sets you free and joy is your natural state.

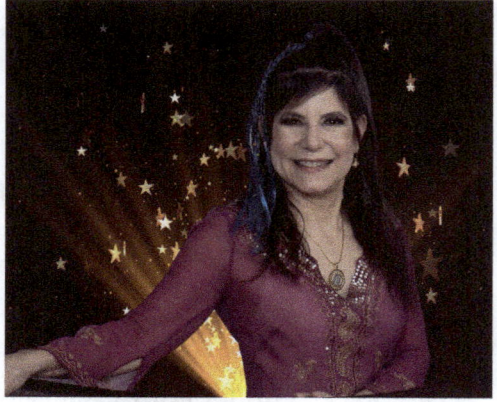

After pouring her heart and soul into caring for three loved ones with terminal illnesses, SueZee's body reached a breaking point. Waking up paralyzed from a debilitating Lupus flare, she faced a daunting crossroad, take the harmful prescription drugs she was handed or continue to suffer. Refusing to surrender to conventional treatments, she listened to her inner guidance and embarked on a courageous quest for alternative solutions. Her odyssey led her to the profound healing power of sound therapy, which not only restored her physical health but also reignited her passion for life.

As the founder of **Acoustic Therapeutix**, a Long Island-based sanctuary for sound healing, and **The Happiness**

Now Network, a movement of joyful living, SueZee is here to help you drop the noise of the world and tune into the music of your soul. Through her transformational sessions, playful improv-infused workshops, and happiness mindset trainings, she helps you break free from limitations, reclaim your light, and dance into the life you were always meant to live—healthy, whole, free and wildly happy.

Because when you align with your soul's frequency of freedom… *everything* is possible.

You can contact SueZee:

https://www.acoustictherapeutix.com

https://www.linkedin.com/in/suezeefinley

https://www.facebook.com/SueZ.Finley

https://www.instagram.com/suezeequest/

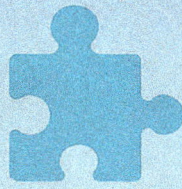

Puzzle Power

Finding Purpose and Potential, Piece by Piece

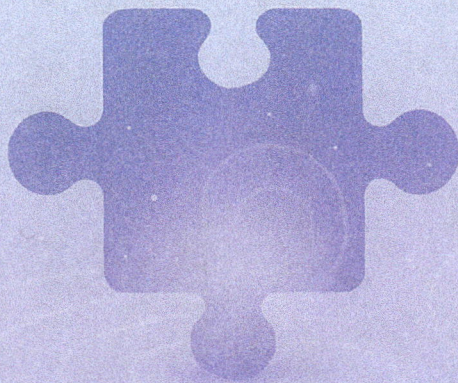

Judy Herman

CHAPTER NINE

PUZZLE POWER:
FINDING PURPOSE AND POTENTIAL, PIECE BY PIECE

Judy Herman

Opening the Box
"You're not living up to your potential."

Those words, spoken by my mom when I was in high school, stung like a slap and have been buzzing in the background of my life ever since. Mother didn't say them in anger, frustration, or disappointment - she aimed them with a certainty that landed and rippled wider than she probably realized.

Ever since her words have influenced my life in ways that I never realized ... until recently. This chapter is the story of that influence.

Piece One: Potential & Possibilities

My mother was the registrar at my high school, which meant she had access to all the students' grades, scores, and test results. In my junior year, after we all took an IQ test, I went to my mother's office and asked if she knew my results.

"Yes, she said, "but I can't tell you without a note from your guidance counsellor." Cue the teenage eyeroll. Okay, so ethically, she wouldn't tell me the score.

"But I will tell you this . . ." Mother looked me straight in the eye and delivered her message quietly and distinctly, "You're not living up to your potential."

I can still feel the sting of that line, and yet she was right. Her words, though dripping with meaning, were not a scolding or lecture. Just a matter of fact, truth. We both knew I could achieve far more in my life. It wasn't that I was lazy or just didn't care. I did very much. But it wasn't my fault – I had yet to piece together the picture of who I was meant to be and what I was meant to live up to.

She wouldn't tell me the number, but she sure let me know the score!

From that moment on, questions hovered over every stage of life and every achievement: high school, college, marriage, motherhood, creative work, travel adventures, and entrepreneurial ventures. *What does it really mean to live up to my potential? How will I know?*

I thought I had built a full and meaningful life, but it still felt unfinished, like a puzzle with a few stubborn missing pieces. I was chasing a version of myself I wanted to become, yet something was always just out of reach as I reinvented myself more times than I can count. I had all these scattered edge-pieces like skills, talents, experiences, and ideas - but no center picture to guide me.

It wasn't until much later that I finally found what was missing. It wasn't a job title or a personal achievement. It wasn't even a bold new idea for a creative money-making project.

It was a decision - a decision to stop trying to fit my pieces into other people's puzzles and start creating my own. *And to help others do the same.*

What follows is an explanation of how puzzles provided purpose and how one woman's words motivated me to finally realize my potential.

✿ Piece Two:
Contents & Portents from My Past

Growing up, I was considered the smart one, articulate and clever - and it felt good when people were impressed with my bright mind and quick wit.

I capitalized on positive first impressions, but to be honest, it came easily to me, without my making much of an effort. Good genes, perhaps, since my dad was very intelligent; at age fourteen, he became the youngest child ever to graduate from Boys' High in Brooklyn, New York.

He succeeded academically because he was smart, but socially and athletically, high school was a disaster for him.

At the time, there were A and B semesters in the public-school year, and my dad was so smart that he skipped all the B semesters. Intellectually, he was mature beyond his classmates, but physically and emotionally, he was very immature compared to his peers.

Dad could forget about competing in the sports arena, which he loved, or playing the dating game to find love. The boys were much older and more mature physically, while no high school girl of 18 was interested in a 14-year-old as a boyfriend.

He graduated an adolescent, not a man.

My father's life experience as a boy came back to haunt him as a parent when I was 6 years old. The elementary school counselor advised that I skip the next grade and go directly to third.

Dad's reaction was so intense that I was shocked by such an unusual emotional upset to his usually even keel. He was emphatically and loudly determined at any cost that I would have a regular school experience with my same age and stage peers, so as not to suffer the same fate that he did by being too smart for his own good.

As a young girl, I wondered if, amid all this upset, it was worth it to be smart. I liked being bright, loved learning, and then teaching what I knew by playing school, with my dolls who were willing, and my little sister who was not. Even then, I knew it was important to be smart, to be true to myself and who I was to become. Years later, I understood the significance of intelligence being one of the key pieces I needed to live up to my potential.

You're allowed to have fun while getting smarter

When I was about nine years old, we visited family friends whose children were teenagers. I was a bit intimidated by those big kids, but fortunately, they introduced me to the board game "Clue", and we started to play. After one round,

I jumped up and declared, "It was Colonel Mustard in the Drawing Room with the rope!"

Mic drop! I was correct on the first guess, and the older players were amazed and praised me, which raised my confidence. I felt empowered and wanted more.

I did get more game competition whenever my parents went out for the evening, and they invited two elderly neighbors, Mrs. Peterson and her niece, Mrs. Walker, to stay with me and my younger sister. We were always excited to see them because it meant a whole evening of playing card games at the dining room table.

The ladies taught us the basics so that we understood how to play, slowly at first to get the concept, building speed and strategy with practice. Competitive Double Solitaire with four decks of cards was a favorite, often fast and furious! I remember being challenged and impressed by the quick play and skill of the "old ladies" who were probably younger than I am now.

Another card game popular in our family was - and still is - *Casino*. It can be played by all ages (I was taught by my grandmother) and two or more players can participate. The basics are simple - you can learn in one round - but it takes strategic skills to win the game and confidence to take a risk.

The concepts I learned playing these games led to techniques I now use in my classes, making sure my students thoroughly understand the basics in the simplest form first, before increasing the difficulty.

Just as there's no jumping in at the deep end when learning to swim, you don't start with the hardest puzzles when learning how to play. Don't try a 1,000-piece jigsaw puzzle of the Milky Way Galaxy as a first attempt puzzle. It's far better to start with a 50-piece puzzle of a Milk Bottle to understand the flow of the game. Once mastered, you can add more pieces to increase the difficulty.

✳ Piece Three: Pathways – When Passion Meets Purpose

I've always loved word games, wordplay, and bantering, which I call "clevering." It's a way to sharpen not just my mind, but my wit and confidence. Through play, I was training my brain and building the cognitive reserve of knowledge I would later depend on.

"I like Words . . . May I Have a Few With You?" That was the title of the very first educational series I did for an experimental project as a sophomore English teacher at Evanston Township High School, just north of Chicago. *It was produced on videotape…* in the late 1960s. We teachers at the highly rated progressive school were pioneers in using this new technology. It was very primitive: I had fun flash cards with simple illustrations of the meanings behind familiar words and phrases used in a course on etymology (the study of the origin of words).

I wish I had a copy of that tape now that I'm back to creating educational videos and Zoom presentations. Today, I present brain games online and in-person classes for good reason - to share them as tools, especially with older adults who might feel anxious about their abilities and need my method, guidance, and encouragement to regain their cognitive confidence.

Even as my adult responsibilities and practical roles increased. I continued to play word games, not just for the fun and mental stimulation, but for the feeling. There's something magical about the moment a scrambled mess of letters transforms into a sentence, or a cryptic clue is revealed. That feeling, that lightbulb moment, is addictive.

After a while I was no longer content with just solving puzzles for myself. I wanted to help others light up as well.

Some clues don't have to be solved - they're meant to be shared.

🧩 Piece Four:
Judy on Jeopardy! Preparation for Puzzle Power

Another tape I wish I had was from the 70s, when I appeared on one of the most popular TV quiz programs of all time. The show is still watched regularly, almost religiously, by millions who tune in to compete against the contestants, play the brain game and learn at the same time. Sounds like **"Brain-tertainment"** to me, but of course I'm asking the question, *"What is Jeopardy!?"*

The studio spotlights were so hot that I remember thinking I would be adding to my nervous perspiration already in progress. I was **"terri-cited"** (feeling terrified and excited at the same time). My heart was beating as loud as the familiar theme music . . . *da da dum, dada da da dum* . . .

I jiggled the buzzer in my hand to make sure it was still there, and that my thumb hadn't gone numb, just as I heard my name announced.

And that was my introduction to the world of Jeopardy!

If you've ever wondered what it's like to be on Jeopardy! let me pull back the curtain: It's part brain marathon, part strategy session, part wardrobe change, and part surreal dream, all happening under the spotlight in front of a live audience, being recorded to broadcast to the world in a few months. Phew -that's a lot to take in!

When I was on the show, Jeopardy! was broadcast from the NBC headquarters at the iconic 30 Rockefeller Plaza Building in bustling mid-town Manhattan. Just being there was exciting, especially coming in by train through Grand Central Station and walking up Fifth Avenue! I lived in Chicago at the time, visiting my parents in New York, enjoying playing the tourist for a change.

I auditioned on a Wednesday morning, along with a dozen or so other eager applicants. We all took a thirty-question qualifying test covering a variety of categories. The only question I remember was *"How many matches are there in a book?"* That was back in the days when people smoked cigarettes with abandon, and I guessed the number of matches was the same as cigarettes in the pack. And I was right! *(So, you don't have to go find a matchbook, the answer is 20.)*

Those of us who passed the test with a score of 25 or more were interviewed individually, and a lucky few like me were selected to appear on the program, with tapings starting the next day! I shivered with excitement and delight, thrilled to come back tomorrow to play the game. I really was going to do this!

Here's something most people don't know: contestants are told to bring a change of clothes. Why? Because *three shows were taped each day*, and the producers didn't want contestants to appear wearing the same outfit on two consecutive days!   *They didn't supply the wardrobe, but they did apply the pressure.*

Thursday morning, extra dress in tow, I was back in the studio, gathered with the other contestants to practice playing Jeopardy! on the stage.   The surreal experience was now becoming very real as we got used to working the buzzer and answering questions with a question! During the afternoon, the set, audience, and host all stayed in place, while the contestants were constantly shuffled in and out of their seats like a high-stakes game of musical chairs.

Later, sitting in the "VIP (very important player) section" of the audience, I watched my fellow competitors playing Game 1, then Game 2, and finally Game 3 - all without me! Like a nervous understudy, I watched the others, wondering how I would fare against them.   One by one, they were eliminated before I even had a chance. Games Over for the day, and I was back on the train.

Friday came, and I was starting to feel like a commuter by now, passing through Grand Central without gawking at its awesomeness anymore. I was back in the audience for Game 1, still not selected to play but carefully observing those who were, since I would probably be competing against one of them

Then, finally, Game 2! My name was called, and it was my turn to stand behind the podium. Heart pounding, I was ready, and it was my Game On! Would my brain perform? And what about my thumb?

Really! You might think that the hardest part would be answering the questions. Nope. ***It's mastering the buzzer!*** You have to time it just right - wait until the host finishes reading the clue aloud and then press. Too early? You're locked out for a crucial fraction of a second. Too late? Someone else beats you to it.

And here's the kicker: *when someone else buzzes in first, you can't get in at all!* Your thumb keeps trying, pressing as if your buzzer's not working. But it is. You're just not fast enough, even if you know the answer.

And it also helps when the category is one that you have some knowledge of, not something obscure or even worse, someone else's specialty (extreme sports, Asian geography, or cartoon Superheroes) or whatever topic you know least about.

Most important, it's *the ability to retrieve information quickly* that pays off on Jeopardy! You may know you know the info, but you must recall it instantly and buzz in first.

To answer quickly in any situation, call upon your cognitive reserve. Withdraw from your mental bank. Many of my answers on Jeopardy! came out of my mouth straight from those saved resources, almost without thinking. (A few times I even surprised myself with what I didn't know I knew.)

You don't need to remember everything. You just need the right clue at the right time.

I got lucky with a few answers because of my reserved knowledge. I knew *that "A flower named for former first lady Eleanor Roosevelt"* was a rose, from her hilariously famous quote:

> *" I once had a rose named after me, and I was very flattered.*
>
> *But I was not pleased to read the description in the catalogue:*
>
> *No good in a bed, but fine up against a wall."*

For the interview, I told a cute story about my little daughter and I watching our favorite shows "Sesame Street" and "Jeppy" together over lunch each day. I joked about how learning from TV was fun for all ages, and it started early in our house.

Little did I know then how important **"Brain-tertainment"** would become much later in life. On Jeopardy! I had to answer with a question. These days, I prefer to ask the questions, brain-boosting ones that help people rediscover what they thought they'd lost.

To be honest, most of my first game was a blur of answers and questions. Yet somehow, we ended up going into Final Jeopardy! with me in the lead. I could actually win! The Final Jeopardy! category was *"Legends of the Wild West!"*

Oh boy, here we go … the only cowboy character I could think of in the moment was the subject of a charcoal portrait I had drawn, depicting Gary Cooper in his role as a famous gunslinger of the Old West. Done in an art class, it was good enough to be framed and thus memorable.

I figured out how much I needed to wager to beat the other contestants and bet the amount, not feeling very confident about the category, still wanting to win. To my utter disbelief (and frankly great relief), the final answer related to the Gunfight at O.K. Corral. *"Who is Wyatt Earp?"* I wrote boldly, hoping I could trust that my calculation for betting was correct.

Turns out, my answer was right, and so was the wager! *"Congratulations! YOU are the new Jeopardy! champion."*

And then came the applause, the handshakes, the congratulations from strangers who suddenly saw me as someone extraordinary. *And I was! I was a Jeopardy! Champion!*

It's hard to describe that feeling. It was an *exhilarating cocktail* of "whew!" "Yay" shock, pride, and "now what?" I was on a great emotional high, but there wasn't time to celebrate my win, so no *Champagne for the Champ* ... I barely had time to change.

Full disclosure: My reign was brief, and it wasn't glamorous.
I spent my 30 minutes of fame as the Jeopardy! Champion in the

Ladies Room!

Remember that change of clothes I brought with me? I had to get ready for the "next day's" taping - happening in half an hour! I quickly transformed from contestant to Champion in a new dress, a different headband, and a brighter shade of lipstick for luck. After a final check and appreciative nod to the mirror, I walked back to the studio, ready to step back into the fray of the next game.

On the way, I realized that *something had shifted* - not just the clothes outside my body but the thoughts inside my head. In a matter of minutes, I had gone from eager player to excited winner to Defending Champion. It felt like I had switched from playing offense to defense at halftime!

It's one thing to win. It's another to defend the title when someone's coming for the crown.

There was one contestant I was hoping not to play against after seeing him in the practice rounds. He was a small man with a big ego, which can be a dangerous combination. So, of course, there he was standing to my left as the iconic theme music began. We were all introduced, and after recognition of me as the current Champion, the categories were revealed. I selected first, answered correctly, and the battle was on.

"Wait - why is my buzzer not working?"

Oh, no! Not again! The cocky little man next to me had just buzzed in ahead of everyone once more, no matter if he knew the answer. He was smart and sneaky. Locking his opponents out by buzzing immediately on every question was the devious strategy used by this cagey fellow to my great disadvantage, because it worked! By the end of Double Jeopardy!, he had accumulated the most points, so he had the upper hand in the game.

Fortunately, I had a good chance against him since I was not far behind going into the Final, where the category was *"Government Agencies."* All right, then, I still had a chance.

Decision time: I thought I might be able to figure out an answer from the clue, so I was tempted to go all in and hope my opponent would get it wrong. Or I could bet nothing, he could still get it wrong, in which case - now came the *mindshift from points to dollars* - I'd end up with more money! If he got the question right and wagered enough, well, then it was his game no matter what I did.

"In the first game, I played to win. In the second, I played not to lose."

Go for it! In the end, I did bet the lot, and he bet just enough to beat me since we both answered correctly, *"What is the F.C.C.?"* Today, I have no clue as to the actual clue, but I was able to figure it out when it counted.

And so, my reign as Jeopardy! Champion was over almost as quickly as it had begun. Late Friday afternoon, heading home on the train with my fellow commuters, I smiled thinking of the whirlwind events of the day. From being an audience member, to challenging contestant to defending champion and back, all in under two hours! However, the details would have to stay within me for a while - I had to keep the outcome a secret until the show aired in mid-August. And it was still June!

On the day the show was broadcast in Chicago, I was finally able to celebrate my win with others. A good friend hosted a "watch party" luncheon in my honor, where, surrounded by supporters, I was hailed as the Jeopardy! Champion of the day. It was great acclaim, but the fun was short-lived. Only I knew what was coming next.

24 hours later, I watched the second game … alone. Besides being fixated on the sneaky tactics of my opponent, I saw where I might have played better (I knew I'd hesitated on a few questions and could have wagered more on the Daily

Double). I felt and absorbed the loss of the game on my own. I was a little sad and still a bit mad, but mostly I was glad that I no longer had to keep the details to myself. I was able to let go of the weight of knowing the outcome once it was out to the world.

Jeopardy! certainly gave me my 30 minutes of fame and a lifetime of bragging rights. The show also taught me the importance of *trusting my knowledge* (Eleanor's rose), *taking a risk* (betting it all on Final Jeopardy!), *and having confidence to succeed* (I brought a change of clothes).

Some further Jeopardy! Takeaways to consider:

Just Knowing the Information Isn't Enough - it's How Quickly you can Recall It.

Confidence and timing can matter more than pure knowledge. You might know the answer, but if you don't buzz in, someone else will. Don't wait until you're "sure"- trust yourself and go for it.

Stay Cool when the Spotlight's Hot

The real test wasn't the trivia - it was staying calm with lights, cameras, and nerves on fire. Your brain works better when you're not in panic mode. *Preparation pays off - and so does staying calm under pressure.*

Your Brain's Been Practicing for this Moment

Jeopardy! didn't teach me facts - it revealed the ones already there. *Your brain is smarter than you give it credit for.* You know more than you think. *Withdraw from the cognitive reserve of information you have in your mental bank.*

Be Ready for Success

I won - and had to change outfits *immediately* for the next game. Be ready to pivot. Always bring a change of clothes*! In reality or metaphorically, be prepared for success every way you can!*

A Single Win Can Rewrite Your Story

Thirty minutes on stage changed how I saw myself forever. **Confidence comes from doing, not just dreaming.** *One step forward can spark a whole new chapter.*

For some simple, practical, easy to apply ways to stay sharp, scan the code for my e-Book, **10 Top Brain-tertainer™ Tips: Improve your Memory Now**

My biggest Jeopardy! takeaway wasn't the money or the title or even the classy Grollier Encyclopedia set I won. It was experiencing the power of entertaining learning. Even if you don't initially know the answer you can learn from the question. From this idea, years later I developed the concept of "Brain-tertainment" featuring entertaining brain games I design with fun in mind.

Now I get to bring the joy of "learning without studying" to others - not with trivia, but with tools to sharpen memory, build confidence and outsmart aging brains, one puzzle at a time. I create word and memory games, puzzles and brain challenges which stimulate different areas of the brain. The program offers something vital: an entertaining way for people to reconnect with their minds, their memories and themselves.

✽ Piece Five:
Possibilities – Clarity, Confidence, & Connection

"I didn't outgrow the puzzle. I outgrew the picture I thought it had to be."

The evolution from game-lover to Jeopardy! champion to the **"Brain-tertainer™"** blends *my personal growth with professional purpose.* Today, helping others build cognitive confidence feels like putting the pieces into place, not just for myself, but for everyone who comes searching for their own "missing pieces."

As with everything, it started with my mother. She began having trouble coming up with a word or remembering the name of the person she'd had lunch with - or even the restaurant where they had eaten. It was very frustrating for Mother, and she would become so anxious in the moment that she couldn't think clearly and lost focus. She berated herself for her shortcomings instead of overcoming them.

I knew my mom liked doing daily word games in the newspaper, particularly the "Jumble" anagram and Word Search puzzles. I started working with her on those, giving some strategies and tips for play. We started simply to really understand the concept of the game. With practice, not only did she get better at the games, *but her confidence in her cognitive ability grew the more she was able to do.*

She wanted to do more. And she did! With my guidance and encouragement, coupled with her enthusiasm, Mother became more competent at the games which increased her confidence and lessened her anxiety about trying something new.

Mother and Me
In the photos we're the same age – looking and feeling great at 78 is in the genes!

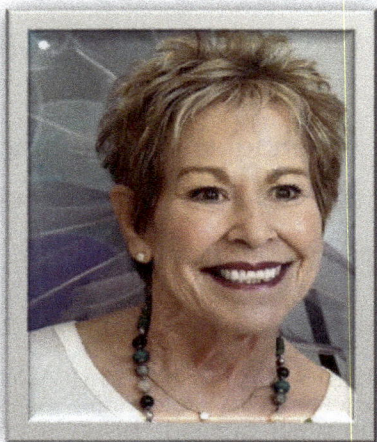

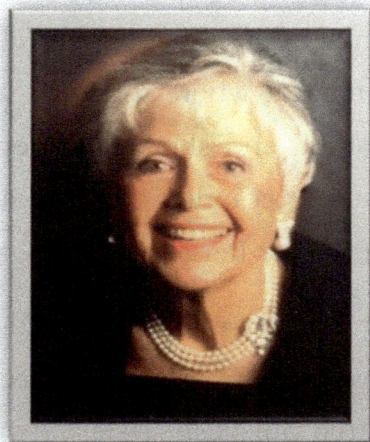

As she got older Mother needed the lifestyle transition from living on her own at a country club in Florida to an independent senior residential community in New Jersey, closer to most of the family. It was the right move to the right place at the right time.

Once she was settled in, I asked the activities director if the community offered a program similar to what I was doing with puzzles. They didn't, but she suggested that I might want to try my method with the other residents. I thought, "I can do that." Having earned a B.S. degree in Education from the University of Wisconsin and having experience as a high school English teacher, I was familiar with creating a lesson plan and comfortable speaking in front of a group.

The next time I visited I'd prepared a presentation – and ended up speaking to a very large group of residents. They were curious, I think, to see my mother's daughter as well as wanting to hear what I had to say.

That first class went so well that afterwards my proud mother came up to me and said enthusiastically, "You were so good! *Nobody fell asleep*! *And nobody left*!" Thus, the bar was set.

I have since come to learn that those words were high praise for a lecturer in senior communities, where dozing off or walking out of a program can be a regular occurrence.

And that's how my *innovative* **"All Aboard the Brain Train"** cognitive fitness program for seniors began. Over the years I've encouraged thousands of students to "keep their minds on track" using puzzles and word games to stimulate different areas of the brain.

The journey got off to a great start when the lovely Program Director, Laura Braff, opened the doors to other Hyatt Classic senior communities by recommending me and my program to her colleagues in South Florida. Thanks to her, for a few years I enjoyed teaching classes not just here but in New York and New Jersey when I visited.

Hello colleagues!

I am so pleased to recommend this fabulous new program presented by a daughter of a resident of ours.

All Aboard the "BRAIN TRAIN", conducted by Judy Herman addresses memory problems, difficulty with words and understanding new concepts in a fun way. Her series will present enjoyable ways to clarify thinking, improve creativity and problem solve. Judy lives in Florida, but visits her mom frequently in New Jersey and will be available to conduct her program at several Classic Residences.

If you are interested in finding out more, please contact her at herman_judy@hotmail.com

Our residents love her – and so do I!

Best regards,
Laura

Laura Braff, Programs Director
Classic Residence by Hyatt
655 Pomander Walk
Teaneck, NJ 07666
201-836-3634, ext. 222
lbraff@hyattclassic.com

From: judy herman [mailto:herman_judy@hotmail.com]
Sent: Monday, August 15, 2005 3:12 PM
To: Braff, Laura
Subject: RE: Classic Residence in Teaneck Recommends "The Brain Train"

Hi, Laura -

Thanks so much for the great references and intros. I know how important your recommendation will be for me to get the Brain Train on the right track with the Classic organization. I will be in touch with the various residences and hope to set up some appointments in the coming week or so. I'll keep you posted on progress "down the line."

I really appreciate that you said such nice things about me and the course, and my mother who is reading along with me is beaming with pride! We're having a good time together here in Florida and send our best love and regards to you.

Judy

Twenty years later I am still teaching classes in 15 different communities each month; Laura and I keep in touch and somewhere I have a copy of the email she wrote back in 2005 that got the Brain Train program on track!

My mother's initial struggle with memory issues became the motivation for a meaningful entrepreneurial journey focused on healthy aging and cognitive engagement for seniors. **"Brain-tertainment"** started to come into focus, not as a concept, but as a calling. I was finally ready to create a way to help others strengthen their minds, find their spark, and feel fully themselves again.

When I stepped fully into my role as the **"Brain-tertainer™"** I began teaching what I loved, sharing the same types of puzzles I had used with my mother - at first to keep her mentally engaged, and eventually, to stay connected as her memory declined. Each class, each workshop, became a tribute to her and a tool for others.

And here's what I learned: every one of us has the power to build cognitive confidence.

You don't need a high IQ, high-tech tools or a perfect memory. You need practice taking small, consistent actions that signal to your brain: "I'm still in here and I'm still learning." I've seen these small actions lead to big transformations. I've seen self-doubt replaced by self-confidence. I've seen people rediscover their voice, their wit, their spark, themselves.

If you're wondering where to start, try some **"Brain-tertainer™"** Tips:

Break your routine. Brush your teeth with your non-dominant hand. Take a different route. Rearrange the kitchen drawer. Your brain lights up when you shake things up.

Play with words. Crossword puzzles, anagrams, and popular online games available free from the New York Times, like *Wordle*, *Connections*, *Strands*, and *Spelling Bee*. Even five minutes a day can improve verbal fluency and short-term memory.

Challenge your recall. Before looking at your calendar, try to name your appointments and activities. Remember phone numbers without your contact list. After watching a movie or reading an article, summarize it to a friend from memory.

Laugh more. It increases oxygen to the brain and releases neurochemicals that enhance learning and make you feel good. Whether or not it's the best medicine, everything's better with a smile.

Begin building your own brain confidence when you scan the code for Neurobic Exercises to do at home - without breaking a sweat!

The Final Piece:
Finishing the Puzzle & Finding the Full Picture

It took me years to realize that I wasn't just missing pieces, I was missing the right perspective. Like one of those hidden picture puzzles, what you see depends on how you view it.

The words, *"You're not living up to your potential,"* weren't about accolades, awards or titles. They were about my ability and my challenge to become the complete person I was meant to be.

My mother wasn't pushing me to achieve more. She was encouraging me to become more. She showed me that potential isn't something you pursue. It's how you live every day, in the way you show up for others to discover their own strengths. She was challenging me to step into something deeper - a life of meaning, connection, and contribution.

I may never know my IQ, but I finally figured out my 'Y'

In a way, working with seniors to sharpen their brains, build self-confidence and outsmart forgetfulness is not just my mission. It's a tribute to the woman who saw my potential before I could. It's my way of saying "Thank you, Mother" as I carry on her legacy, one active brain, one stimulating puzzle, one confident "aha!" moment at a time.

Helping others outsmart forgetfulness and creating confidence in their ability turned out to be the very thing that helped ME live up to MY potential. Not by impressing anyone, but by empowering them. Not by chasing the spotlight, but by lighting the way for someone else.

There is a Japanese concept called *"Ikigai"* (pronounced ee-key-guy) that combines the terms *iki* meaning "alive" or "life," and *gai*, meaning "benefit" or "worth." In other words, it's the idea of finding your personal purpose in life.

"The final piece wasn't missing after all. It was just waiting for me to place it with purpose."

And wouldn't you know it? Once I had my focus, *the picture on the box started to become clear.* My love for language and learning. My passion for performance. My craving to connect, entertain, educate and encourage. Everything came into place as the pieces came together.

For all the titles I've held, the roles I've played, and the places I've been, becoming the **"Brain-tertainer™"** feels truest to who I am. All those years of puzzles, games, teaching, speaking - they weren't hobbies. They were clues pointing me toward my purpose, my Why, my "Ikigai."

I am now living up to my potential by helping others achieve theirs.

❋ It was the final piece my mother always knew I would find.

To end with some **"Brain-tertainment"** for you, here's an example of an anagram game I call "The Word Wheel," which is always very popular in my presentations. The word that uses all the letters is relevant to the theme of my chapter.

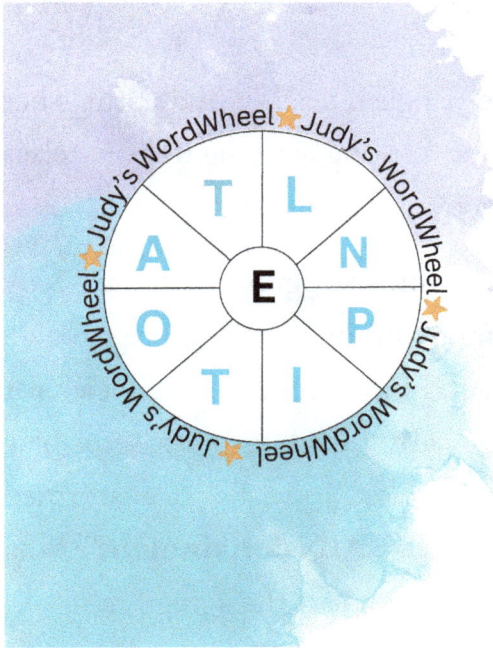

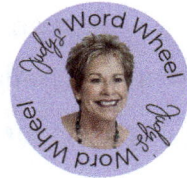

Make as many words as you can from the letters in the wheel.
Use each letter only as many times as it appears in the puzzle. Do not double.

YOU MUST USE THE LETTER IN THE CENTER OF THE CIRCLE IN EVERY WORD FOR IT TO COUNT

There may be others, but they don't count in this game.
Proper nouns, plurals, foreign words and abbreviations do count.

Words can be **any length**, and there is a **9-letter word using all the letters!**

Answer: The 9-letter word is

POTENTIAL

About the Author

Judy Herman, **the "BRAIN-tertainer™,"** is an entertaining speaker, engaging educator and Cognitive Confidence Coach. She supports adults concerned about age-related cognitive decline, helping them to stay sharp and mentally active.

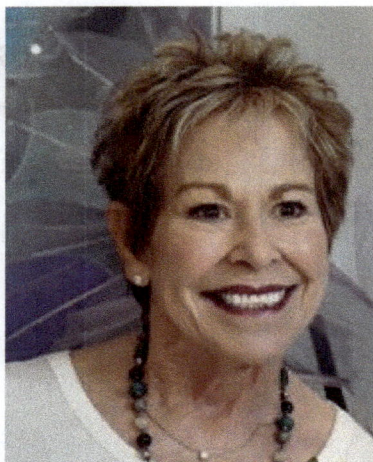

As a **Jeopardy! Champion,** puzzle enthusiast and former English teacher, Judy brings her love of language, laughter, and lifelong learning to every class and audience she meets, in person and online.

Motivated by her own mother's cognitive decline, Judy created her signature "learning without studying" approach, using puzzles, word games, and brain-boosting strategies for Boomers and savvy seniors. By blending purposeful play with practical memory techniques, Judy has transformed traditional brain training into **"BRAIN-tertainment"™** a fun, fresh, and inspiring way to outsmart the aging brain.

Inspired by her mother's encouragement to reach her full potential, for the past two decades Judy has entertained and empowered other seniors to achieve greater confidence and a renewed sense of possibility. She has travelled the world and after living in New York, Chicago, and London, Judy now happily resides in Delray Beach, Florida, where she looks forward to spending the "next best rest of her life," fulfilling her purpose and encouraging others to do the same.

To schedule a presentation, class, individual or group coaching session:

phone: 561-542-7830

e-mail: *judy@braintertainer.com*

For more information, visit *www.thebraintertainer.com*

Check out Judy's free e-book **"Top Ten Tips for Memory Improvement"**

https://brain-tertainer.ck.page/top-tips

Top 10 Braintertainer Tips ebook

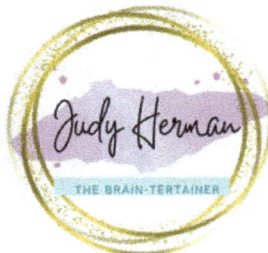

THE BRAIN-TERTAINER

IT'S A GREAT DAY FOR ICE CREAM

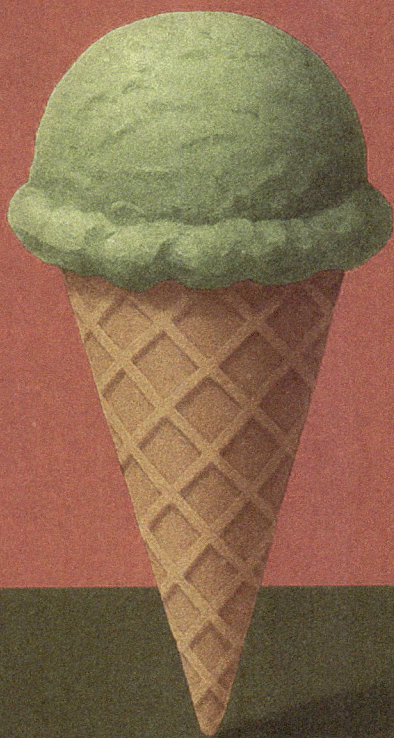

JACKY FOSS

3 beautiful souls have impacted my life enabling me to share my story.

Scully my fur baby RIP June 2007- April 2025

Paddy my soul mate, my husband, my reason for sharing my work

Kat my oldest friend in this lifetime. You have always seen me, loved me, accepted all of me.

CHAPTER TEN

IT'S A GREAT DAY FOR ICE CREAM

Jacky Foss

The Art of Conversation

Sitting, waiting, people watching to pass the time

Going through multiple conversations in my head

Questioning, arguing with the decline of all verbal interactions

Outwardly smiling at strangers hoping they receive my gesture with grace and take it further in their day

Feeling a spring to my step unsure if it is my nerves creating a space for the return of my anxiety or the feeling of being praised

I really want to continue but I have other tasks that need to be executed

As I run through my to do list the silent promises in my head are taking up more space

Digging deep into my heart I want to show the art of conversation is still relevant

An Apple a Day

But the rooms inside of my head are being filled with unwanted thoughts and preparations for crisis meetings

Struggling with the concept of break glass in case of an emergency

Frantically searching, pleading for anyone to catch my eyes

Hoping someone will see my pain, offer a hand, a chair anything to prevent me from falling down again

Blacking out, laying still unsure of what awaits me

Voices in the distance accompanied by sirens and earth-shattering screams

This is not how I envisioned my day

Ending up in emergency trying to explain I am not crazy just struggling with a little pain

Please I plead no medications or restraints

All I am craving is some meaningful conversations to get me through my days.

© By JM FOSS

Let your Light Shine

We all have a story inside us waiting to be shared, waiting for someone to give us permission to share our innermost and deepest thoughts. Give us permission to step outside of the box we have placed ourselves in so we can survive. So we can control and maintain a persona that has become more real than anything we have known or experienced.

I get to share part of my story with you. Why only part of my story? Because my story is a never-ending journey, one that is always evolving, always changing, and always looking for a different ending.

I am the youngest of 4 girls, and we grew up in the country, attending a school that had less than 20 students. After moving to a secondary school with more than 400 students to finish my high school journey, at a school of 3,500 students... needless to say, this didn't end well. I got in trouble for forging my mum's signature on my notes to explain my absence from class because I believed I never belonged. I had no real friends, and thought I had no real purpose but to sit in a room and take up space. Then, in my final year, I just signed my own name on any notes. Problem fixed.

Sports day was one of my favourite activities at school. Running track brought me joy, excitement, freedom, and an opportunity to escape. I broke athletic records and made the South Island Championships of New Zealand, which still to this day brings a smile to my face. In these moments, I felt free. No judgment, no fear, just the butterflies in my stomach cheering me on.

Upon reflection, it seems I was always running from something. Running from my current reality or trying to escape my very loud and busy mind. You see, my mind never shuts off—there is always an internal chatter, offering impertinent opinions and self-destructive thoughts. Negative chatting about how I should be quieter, I should be smarter, I should… always with the. "I shoulds." Never a "Great job! You smashed it today." Never "You are making a difference, and you matter." Only negative noise.

From my late teens to my early twenties, I was subject to constant mental torment from someone with whom I was in a relationship. Daily hearing that you aren't smart enough, you aren't pretty enough, you aren't thin enough—it all played nicely into my insecurities, causing me to spin into my own pit of darkness. The kind of darkness that offers no warmth, no security… just never-ending dread.

Being in my early twenties and working long hours trying to please everyone, being "that" person everyone could rely on and see me as an asset, was a perfect fit for the next chapter in my life. Coming out of a toxic relationship and being unhealed, I stepped into another relationship and went on rinse and repeat. The mental torment deepened, and I allowed myself to go further into that dark pit of dread.

The more I threw myself into work and accommodated the needs of others, always doing anything that took the focus away from me and how I was feeling the more I struggled. It got so bad that one day, I slid down the wall at work. Paralysed, unable to speak, just staring into space and wondering what has become of my life. Upon reflection, I felt as though I was taking up space and not contributing to anything of value. The world I was living in didn't match the world outside of me. So many years of feeling isolated, different, and insufficient were taking their toll on my mind, body, and soul.

The stories we tell ourselves can be heavy, soiled, destructive, and, in hindsight, not true. But these are our stories that our mind tricks us into believing as our truth. What really happened in my mind and what played out in reality is subjective to the viewer.

What I can share with conviction is I was ashamed of not being able to do it all. Who would believe a healthy, active 22-year-old is mentally struggling? I had a roof over my head, food in my stomach, clothes on my back, a job, and my freedom. What would people say if I reached out for help? Would they even listen? Would they even care? The "what if" game was easier to play than stepping up and placing myself in another vulnerable position.

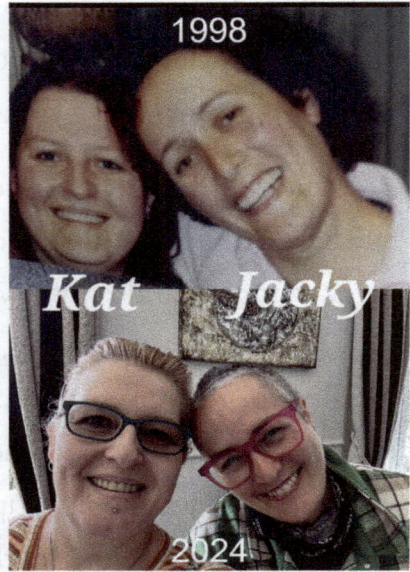

Over and over in my mind I could hear the voices of others, saying, "What do you have to be sad about?" "You are one of the happiest people I know!" "If you get sad, then what hope is there for us?"

To that 22-year-old me, I'm sorry. I'm sorry I couldn't help you. I'm sorry I didn't have the strength to ask for help. I'm sorry I chose over and over to push my boundaries and ignore my triggers, which kept on causing you more pain and pushed you further into the dark void. I'm sorry I never chose you!

Days, weeks, and months merged into one long foggy existence. Nothing had changed. I still felt overwhelmed, insecure, and was in constant battle with myself. It wasn't until I was found at the top of my friend's parents' wardrobe that there was a shift in my circumstances. This should have been an invitation for me to reach out and ask for help to escape this internal prison I had created for myself. Should have and could have never had been much help.

Eventually, through some kind of miracle and the unwavering support of my friend Kat, who has always seen my light and accepted me for all my quirks and misgivings, gave me the strength to muster up the courage to go to the Doctor and ask for help. In my mind, I had convinced myself that nothing was wrong, and I was being overly dramatic; it was just crying, being fatigued, and in what some would call a deep depression that was just a phase. Cutting down on my hours and trying to get more sleep will improve my mood, and if I just adjusted my attitude, I would be fine in a couple of days. After all, I am a healthy 22-year-old who doesn't have anything to complain about… right?

While sitting in the Doctor's office waiting to be seen, I was questioning why I was even here. I didn't need help, just a few early nights and I will be fine. No need to waste the Doctor's time or my money. But just as I was about to get up out of my chair and leave, my name was called. Shit! Maybe if I ran right now, surely, they couldn't catch me? But dutifully, I followed the nurse back to the room.

Sitting opposite the Doctor, I explained what was happening and how I couldn't understand why I wasn't Wonder Woman. "Why couldn't I do everything I felt I needed to and function at a level that was deemed ok and sustainable to my health? Seriously, why wasn't I able to cope? I'm 22 years of age. Young, otherwise healthy, easy-going, but a little neurotic, and a hardworking people pleaser. Again," I asked the Doctor, "Why couldn't I cope?"

The Doctor said something of value, I'm sure. Honestly, I don't recall what was said because I was in a fog of unknowns. What I do recall is being given a script for Prozac and directions on how to take it and—importantly—to seek medical advice before stopping medication.

The next 3 months I was wrought with guilt, fear, uncertainty, and more shame. The shame and what-ifs outweighed any positive changes the medication could offer, and the shame of having to go back to the Doctor and share my updates and experiences since starting the medication and reliving the same story over and over wasn't high on my to-do list. The shame of going to the pharmacy to fill my script. What if someone I knew saw me? What if the pharmacist wanted to ask me questions? Again, the what-ifs outweighed any positive changes the medication could offer.

So, the only thing I could do was to stop taking the medication. And that is what I did. I didn't listen to my doctor's advice about seeking medical advice before stopping my medication. Seriously, I'm 22-years-old. What possibly could go wrong?

There were countless times I'm sure I wanted to scream out for help. Act out a little like a child and have a tantrum so someone would notice and ask me if I was ok, ask me if I needed help, ask me anything! Anything that resembles an act of kindness, an acknowledgement that "I see you and you're not alone." To tell me I am safe. To tell me everything's ok.

Deciding to leave my home country of New Zealand in 1999 to move to Australia was a decision made on a whim. I was originally going to Tasmania, Australia, for a 10-day tour that would take me on my first solo trip overseas. It was only a few weeks before I was due to depart, I received the news that I was the only person who had booked this tour, and this being the case meant it was cancelled. So, what was I going to do? It was decided I would go to Brisbane and stay with some family friends for 10 days. Then out of nowhere, my boyfriend at the time said, "Go to Brisbane and I'll be there in 6 weeks. We can start a new adventure together". That is what I did. I quit my job, sold my belongings, stood at the airport crying and wondering what I had just gotten myself into.

Moving to Australia, I could be forgiven for thinking that my life would get better. The depression would subside, and the loneliness and insecurity of being me would be a thing of the past. The part of me I was running from would stay on the tarmac back in New Zealand as the plane took off to my new, exciting, anything other than what I might have right now, life.

Landing in a new country had its excitement and the promise of more opportunities than I could poke a stick at. Still, I couldn't silence the escape plan I had swirling around in my head. It was becoming apparent that no matter how far I travelled, I couldn't run away from the one thing that scared me more than anything else in the world... I couldn't run away from me!

The mind chatter, negative thoughts, and insecurities increased 10-fold being in another country. No matter how many letters I would write home to family and friends, sharing my adventures, about any upcoming events, or the antics of trying to escape spiders the size of dinner plates, it couldn't numb the internal and external voices I was battling with daily. I reminded myself that nobody wants to hear that you are so homesick, but almost every day, I wished I could come home, come back to the familiar streets that provided safe passage to escape your mind.

The place where I could hide and be seen in the light that was comfortable for everyone but me. I was playing a part after all. It was too late to turn back now. Too late to admit I was wrong to leave my home country for what I thought could provide the solace I was craving. I thought it would provide a better hiding place for my shame and guilt I was carrying, being a 22-year-old having a breakdown. The shame and guilt of being me.

My time in Australia provided me with some exceptional experiences, but finding my feet and a way to escape my very core was exhausting and soul-destroying. Every day, I would wake up and wonder what game I would be playing today or who I would be playing with. Hide and *NOT* Seek was always one of my top games.

I was on the edge of collapsing into the dark void that no matter where I found myself, always called my name, and each day it was getting stronger, louder, and more persistent. This voice was the most constant thing in my life and, on some level, provided me with a sense of love and kindness I was craving. All I needed to do was to surrender. Surrender everything, and the dark void would take care of the rest.

In the early 2000s, that's what I did. I chose to see who or what was knocking at my door. I took a deep breath and flung that door open and welcomed the dark stranger whom I knew all too well. The stranger whose name I never wanted to speak out loud. The stranger who in fact was my best friend, known to many and me as… depression.

There was nothing special about that day. There is no particular reason why I decided to surrender to depression and the false promises of a better life for me and others if I left this place permanently. Nothing special indeed. Until there was.

I went to work to clear out my desk and complete any outstanding tasks. Ironic that even at my darkest moment, I was still being that people pleaser, still trying to erase my presence. The self-hatred, guilt, and shame never took a backseat even after I had surrendered everything and done everything that was asked of me. It was bloody relentless!

Was it the fact I didn't have to care anymore or the promise of peace that I asked a very close friend to have lunch with me one last time? Mr. E was a kind soul, softly spoken, well-dressed, intelligent, and always wore the most intoxicating cologne. As we sat in the park chatting, admiring the surrounding beauty and people watching, he turned to me and asked me if I was ok. The way his words penetrated my whole body made me feel flushed and lightheaded. What was happening? What was I feeling? Why was I feeling this now? Surely, he is just asking out of politeness. Surely, he can't see the dark void inside of me. Surely, he doesn't see the true me. The me that is screaming out for love, kindness, and compassion. The true me that doesn't want to surrender to my depression.

Mr. E sitting there with tenderness and compassion in his eyes, staring at me, waiting but not pushing me for an answer that I believed he already knew. An answer of omission, I am not ok. Sitting there wringing my hands and trying to hold back tears I spoke a voice I had not recognized, speaking with a level of desperation and hope, I blurted out what I knew he had already sensed. I was done. Not just with that day, but with every day that had been and every day that would follow this one. I was done being me. This was my final chapter. No happy ending. No rewrites. One-way ticket to the afterlife. No refunds or date exchanges. Window seat all the way, please.

Even as I write this, I can still feel Mr. E hand resting on top of mine and ever so gently saying "Don't leave." As he pulled me into his arms for the first time, I felt the compassion and kindness I had been craving. I felt my soul become lighter and through my tears all the shame, judgement, and guilt started to shift.

Allowing my mind to empty, I was able to hear the quiet whispers in my soul. No longer the echoes of despair I was starting to experience a thirst for answers to questions I never knew existed. I had spent years suffocating in a cycle of my own haunting thoughts of despair, darkness and suicidal impulses. Now was the time to connect with my inner child and go on an adventure of self-discovery and let curiosity and wonderment lead the way. It was time to be the author of my own story. No more pleasing people. No more being anything but me.

As I delved deeper into spiritual practices, ancient teachings, healing practices, and personal introspection, I discovered a hidden spring of healing. The supernatural wasn't just about mystical forces or unexplained phenomena; it became a gateway to understanding the unseen parts of myself, the parts that had been buried under layers of grief, fear, and self-doubt. The more I allowed myself to embrace this newfound connection to something greater, the more I began to shed the weight of the dark thoughts that had once felt like my only companion.

It was in the quiet moments of stillness, when I looked beyond the surface of my pain and into the mysteries of existence, that I found my soul reaching out. Slowly but steadily, this thirst began to guide me towards my healing journey. It reminded me that there was more to life than my suffering, more to me than the broken pieces I thought I had become. The supernatural, in all its forms, taught me to embrace the unknown, to trust in forces larger than myself,

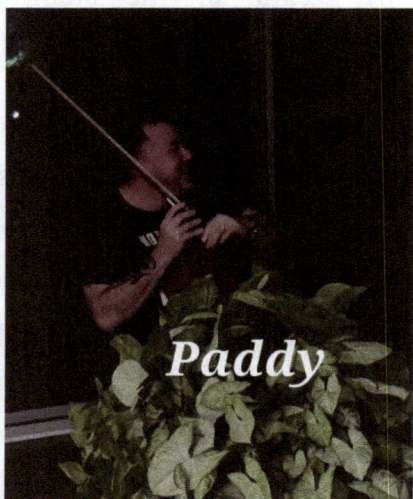

Paddy

and to recognize that even in my darkest hours, there was light waiting to be uncovered.

I began to step into a new chapter of my life. Not one defined by the weight of my past, but one infused with the possibility of transformation, healing, and rebirth. And with each step, I found that the path of healing was not linear, but more layered with mysteries, moments of wonder and a deeper connection to the universe and myself.

Rediscovering my thirst for the knowledge of the universe, healing and discovering the part I was to play, I started to find the strength to open my heart and mind to the possible opportunities that waited for me. Ending the cycle of toxic relationships and accepting my own worth, and starting to accept the idea of having self-love, I found the kind of love that could have come out of a fairytale. This person saw and embraced all my quirks, insecurities, and accepted me for the being I was and any version that would arise. This person is my beautiful husband, Paddy.

Paddy had a 3-legged dog named Harley, and only 3 months after meeting Paddy, I told Harley I was going to marry her Daddy one day and she had to promise not to tell him. Harley kept her promise and in 2007 I married her Daddy in a garden ceremony. Even though she couldn't be with us (she had passed a few years before), we still included her and all our fur babies Oscar, Poo Poo, and Angie in our wedding vows.

Having the support of Paddy I was able to continue my spiritual journey for healing and discovering my true soul purpose. This allowed me to grow deeper in my connection to my inner self and the universe. With guidance from a network of like-minded individuals who uplifted and inspired me I was empowered to release past wounds and embrace a path of transformation. This led to Paddy, Scully (our Jack Russell who is now 17.5 years old), and I to head back home to New Zealand in November 2022, which set me on a trajectory of deeper healing, self-discovery and the beginning of finding my tribe.

In 2023, I discovered the profound power of forgiveness, not only for others but, perhaps most importantly, for myself. I began to understand that forgiveness is a healing balm for the soul, releasing me from the burdens of resentment and anger. It was through this process that I learned to see beyond the illusions created by others—the beliefs, expectations, and judgments that had once been imposed on me. These were not truths, but projections of their own inner struggles and limitations.

By seeing through these veils, I liberate myself from the emotional chains and mental fatigue that had bound me, reconnecting with the essence of who I truly am. I embraced freedom, reclaimed the lost fragments of myself, and found peace in the process. I gave myself permission to love every part of who I am, including the parts that once felt broken or unworthy. This was not always a positive experience. There were days when I wished I could go back to not remembering. Because with every action comes responsibility to be a better person today than you were yesterday. Healing is necessary for growth and expansion, but it can also be a very lonely trip. Be patient with and kind to yourself. Every day is a gift waiting to be opened and enjoyed.

2023 also illuminated the hidden light within me. As I journeyed inward, I connected to the divine spark that resides within every soul. This inner light became my guiding force, helping me navigate through life with some clarity and purpose. After many sleepless nights, I was able to stand in my power and say enough is enough. I will no longer accept others' perceptions of the world as my truth. I uncovered strengths within me that had been dormant for so long, revealing a source of courage, resilience, and wisdom that I had not fully acknowledged before.

It was as if I was awakening to my full potential, stepping into a power I never knew I possessed. Into a power I still wasn't sure I was worthy of or had the capacity to harness. With this newfound strength, I was able to show deeper compassion and kindness, not only towards others but also towards myself. I learned to approach each moment with love and understanding, recognizing that every interaction and every experience was an opportunity for growth.

This year was not just about personal growth; it was a spiritual awakening. I found that true growth comes when we surrender to the process of healing, trusting that every experience, no matter how challenging, is part of a larger divine plan. Through the trials and triumphs, I learned to align with the rhythm of my soul, embracing both the light and the shadows within.

2023 became a transformative year, guiding me toward a deeper understanding of myself and my place in the universe. It was a year that helped me realize that healing is not a destination, but an ongoing journey, one where self-love, forgiveness, and compassion lead the way.

2023 revealed my blueprint for what was to take place in the coming years. Having what I had learnt and experienced in 2023 provided a more stable footing for what was about to erupt in 2024. Let the games begin.

Then 2024 arrived and the games began. No big opening ceremony with fans on the sidelines screaming my name and holding signs of inspiration or encouragement. Nope this was a game for one player. No reset button. No, turning the game off and back on. No backing out. Time to buckle up and surrender to the unknown.

I started the year out feeling confident and very inspired and believing I had it all sorted. I was the only player after all. What could possibly go wrong?

I had just come off a year of spiritual growth and expansion and had decided to quit paid employment and go on a deeper journey of healing and step into the possibility of starting my own healing business. Unknown to me what was about to happen wasn't so much about me offering healings to others as it was to heal those wounds that were buried so deep that it would take me on a path of healing generations of trauma just so I could breathe again.

In January 2024, Paddy and I went away for a week's holiday down south to reset and catch up with my beautiful friend Kat of 30 years. Seeing Kat after so many years of being apart brought back those memories of being found in the top of her parents wardrobe all those years ago. Being with Kat was a bittersweet moment. Here I was standing in front of this beautiful human being who stood by me through my darkest hours and not once judged me or put any expectations on me. And in the same moment I was transported back to one of the darkest periods of my life. Feeling, seeing and hearing my internal screams. As it has always been with Kat and I were able to put that insecure part of me who was found broken all those years ago to rest. How? Through the one thing Kat and I do the best. Laugh. I mean real belly laughs. The kind of laughing you do and nearly wet your pants laughing. During this week, I was able to explore my limits and push past them. I drove the Crown Range from Queenstown over to Wanka and then a few days later drove from Cromwell over the Devil's Staircase to Invercargill to see Kat and then down to Bluff the bottom of the South Island where we celebrated our journey with hot chips before returning to Cromwell—all in one day! I have never done this much driving before, and having Paddy by my side gave me the confidence to keep going.

After all the work, healing, growth and acceptance of myself and others I thought 2024 would be a walk in the park. I would take some time to rest and step into the next chapter of being paid for sharing my gifts.

I had this idea that I would give myself February to reset and then dive right into my new life of spiritual freedom and exploration of the soul. Funny how things don't always turn out the way you want or expect. It is easier for me to reflect and share with you 12 months later because I have lived, experienced, crumbled, cried, and wanted to give up more time I can remember, and yet, here I am.

I spent 2024 delving deep into healing not only me, my ancestors and past lives all for the goal of being a better person, finding my purpose and more importantly finding peace.

I wasn't prepared for the rollercoaster ride I was taking myself on. Around every corner I would be presented with more challenges and questions I either didn't understand or have the strength to find the answers. The healing, the learning, and releasing of trauma just didn't stop. After all the work I had done to this point, I thought "Surely, it must be my turn to shine?"

Over the following months I invested in course after course trying to find answers and make sense of what I was going through. All these courses had value… just some more than others.

The three courses and one process that helped me project deeper and further into my spiritual journey and crack open my heart were:

Medicine Woman Centre for Shamanic and Esoteric Studies - Certificate in Rite of the Six Moons

Esoteric Hypnosis Training Academy - HypnoSuccess Soul Coach

Authentic Education - Difference Maker Acceleration

Akashic Readings for multiple past lives and healing sessions to integrate the lessons that were presented

The Certificate in Rite of the Six Moons connected me to all my bodies: mental, physical, emotional, and spiritual. Through this process, I was able to connect with my ancestors on a deeper level that was required to face, heal and release generations and lifetimes of trauma, all with compassion and respect. This course was a process undertaken over 6 months and required daily ingestion of teaching essences, journaling, and sharing insights online.

Completing my HypnoSuccess Soul Coaching training opened my mind to working in conjunction with my soul and embracing my true soul purpose to be of service. Every time I put my learnings into practice, my soul became more alive and the light within me started to shine brighter, enabling my path to become clearer. Completing this training I have been able to connect with soul and form a relationship of both respect and trust.

Difference Maker Acceleration blew me apart. No more hiding and no more playing the part of victim in my breakdown when I was 22. You see up to this point I hadn't really healed the trauma or released the attachments of shame and guilt even though I had done so much work on myself. Speaking out about burnout

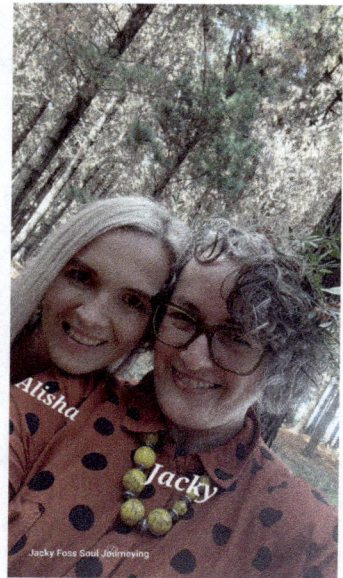

and the mental toll it takes cracked my heart wide open to rid any old patterns and scars to be honoured and released.

Akashic Readings completed by Daniela Birch and Healings by Alisha Robinson and Melissa Garnier brought clarity that I never knew existed. Having a deeper understanding of where my soul had ventured before and the trials and tribulations my soul faced brought both comfort and reassurance and peace to my humanself.

2024 was a year filled with abundant opportunities—opportunities to try new things, gain new skills, and explore emotions I had long ignored or dismissed. I embraced vulnerability and allowed myself to feel deeply, realizing that emotions are not to be feared but welcomed as teachers and healers. By doing so, I started to release the emotional baggage that had been weighing me down and stepped into a state of emotional freedom and balance. Each experience became a lesson, a stepping-stone on my path to self-discovery. With every tear shed, smiles that turned into laughter and every dark thought that was able to turn into a bright light reaffirmed my desire to be of service. To stand in my

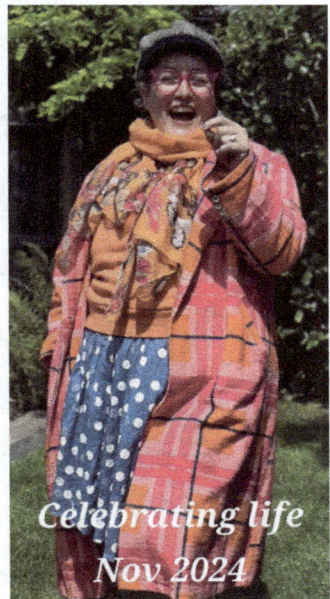

Celebrating life Nov 2024

truth and help others to reach their potential and to make sure no being wakes up feeling alone and lost.

My Key Takeaways from 2024

➢ Never give up on finding your tribe.

➢ Achieving balance is essential for creating harmony and shifting from supporting others to embracing and celebrating your own journey.

➢ Never underestimate the power of healing.

➢ Celebrate the small wins.

➢ Not everyone is going to be excited for you and what your vision and mission entails. This is ok. Once you find your mission and understand why your path becomes clearer.

➢ It's OK to say NO.

➢ Find more JOY in everyday moments.

➢ Taking time to reflect and celebrate all I have done and continue to do isn't being selfish.

If you had told me at the beginning of 2024 what my year was going to be like and how much healing I was going to do. I would have said no thanks. Find someone else for the job.

Don't be scared to share your story. Embrace all the hard and sticky moments as opportunities to grow and evolve.

Finishing 2024 I still had some thoughts about if I had done the right thing.

➢ Getting off the hamster wheel.

➢ Leaving the security of paid employment.

➢ Diving deep into healing myself.

➢ Investing in me to grow and expand as a person and in my new business.

Then today January 1st, 2025, I received my confirmation. I got to be there for my beautiful hubby Paddy to support him in his first cello gig in 2025.

If you are feeling unsure if you are on the right track, look around you. The answers are everywhere.

Embrace all your quirks and lean into being the best version of you. Everyone else is taken.

Everyday is a great day for ice-cream.

Words are My Freedom

Words are my freedom, an extension of me

Words are my light amongst the darken shadows that reside inside of me

Words are my escape from the highway of screams plaguing me

Words are my connections to all that inspires within me

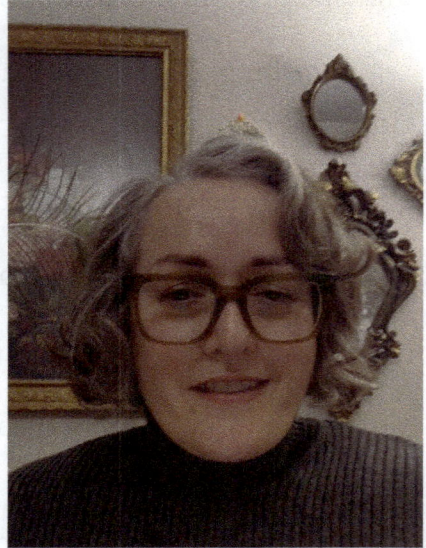

Words are my opportunity to flee

To flee from the inner demons, danger of self-destructive memories

Words are my mighty swords to combat the armies that stand in front of me

Words are my hero's that have the strength to break free

Break free from judgement, disconnect and misery

Words are my fighter jets that light up the skies, enabling the villages below to step out of the darkness, giving them permission to shine

Words are my music that sing my melody

Words are my foundations for the rules and regulations I bestowed upon me

Jacky Foss

Words are my treasures maps where X marks the spot

Words are my very own miracle

Words are my everything

From sunrise to sunset with everything in between

My words are my freedom, my lifeline

My words are my gift from me to you

For your words are your freedom

All you need to do is open the door allowing what's needed to come through.

© By JM FOSS

About the Author

I am Jacky Foss, and I am no longer in a box—I take up space. By throwing out the rule book, I found enchantment in expression. Crafting this bio is not a formality—it's a journey. I invite you to walk with me.

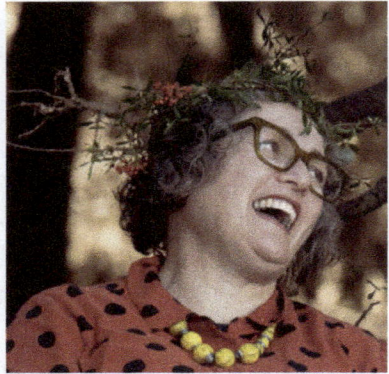

I've worn many hats: nurse, recruiter, manager, and even a Coles team member. But my true passion simmered beneath it all—food. That love birthed a Recipe for Your Soul. Leaving the 9–5 grind wasn't the end. It was the beginning. A blessing disguised as a question: Who am I, really? Working on myself, embracing my individuality— I realized it was never a curse. It was my calling. I stopped building boxes and started creating space. Space to feel. To fear. To be. From that space, a new medium was born: Empowerment Poetry. Together, we explore what's been buried deep for centuries. Through my words, I help you journey through your power. Words are my medium. Words are my freedom. And I'm here—taking up space, unapologetically.

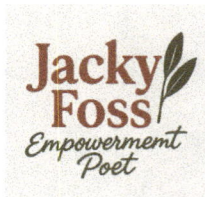

Conclusion

May You Remember

Kristine Skiff, CEO Gift an Author Publishing

If you've made it to this page, then take a breath.

Not a shallow one —

But a deep, real, "I'm-still-here" kind of breath.

You've walked with us through stories of grief, resilience, healing, and homecoming. You've met practitioners who found their power by first losing it. You've seen how healing is never a single moment, but a thread we keep weaving into our lives again and again.

We—every author in these pages—have been in the dark places too. We know the overwhelm of unanswered questions, the exhaustion of being the strong one, the quiet ache of wondering if you'll ever feel whole again. We've lived in doctor's offices and hospital waiting rooms, in prayer and panic, in "what now?" and "what if?" And we've learned that healing isn't found by running faster. It begins the moment we finally stop and listen.

You don't have to earn the right to wellness. You don't have to be perfect, or positive, or productive to be worthy of healing. You already are.

Right now. As you are.

Messy. Magnificent. Mid-process.

Worthy.

And your voice? Your story? It matters more than you know.

You were never meant to disappear behind a diagnosis.

You were never meant to carry it all alone.

If this book has done one thing, may it be this:

May it remind you that your story isn't over.

You are not too late. You are not too broken.

You are not invisible.

We see you.

We believe in your healing.

And if you ever feel your voice slipping away, come back to these pages. Let them hold space for you until you can speak again.

Kristine Skiff

A Traditional Celtic Blessing

May you recognize the light in your own soul.

May your body be a place of peace.

May your mind find its rhythm again.

May you trust the quiet wisdom within.

May love walk beside you, always.

And when the path feels heavy,

May you remember:

You are never walking alone.

www.ingramcontent.com/pod-product-compliance
Lightning Source LLC
Chambersburg PA
CBHW050338270326
41926CB00016B/3509